# THE INTELLIGENT BODY

# THE INTELLIGENT BODY

## REVERSING CHRONIC FATIGUE AND PAIN FROM THE INSIDE OUT

Kyle Davies

Foreword by Gabor Maté

W.W. NORTON & COMPANY

INDEPENDENT PUBLISHERS SINCE 1923

NEW YORK LONDON

For information about permission to reproduce selections from this book,
write to Permissions, W. W. Norton & Company, Inc.,
500 Fifth Avenue, New York, NY 10110

For information about special discounts for bulk purchases, please contact
W. W. NortonSpecial Sales at specialsales@wwnorton.com or 800-233-4830

Manufacturing by Edwards Brothers Malloy
Production manager: Christine Critelli

Library of Congress Cataloging-in-Publication Data

Names: Davies, Kyle L., author.
Title: The intelligent body : reversing chronic fatigue and pain from the
inside out / Kyle L. Davies.
Description: First edition. | New York : W.W. Norton & Company, [2017] |
Includes bibliographical references and index.
Identifiers: LCCN 2016047323 | ISBN 9780393712056 (hardcover)
Subjects: LCSH: Medicine and psychology. | Emotions--Physiological aspects.
| Mind and body. | Healing.
Classification: LCC R726.5 .D37 2017 | DDC 610.1/9--dc23 LC record
available at https://lccn.loc.gov/2016047323

W. W. Norton & Company, Inc., 500 Fifth Avenue, New York, N.Y. 10110
www.wwnorton.com

W. W. Norton & Company Ltd., 15 Carlisle Street, London W1D 3BS

1 2 3 4 5 6 7 8 9 0

**Important Note:** *The Intelligent Body* is intended to provide general information on the subject of health and well-being; it is not a substitute for medical or psychological treatment and may not be relied upon for purposes of diagnosing or treating any illness. Please seek out the care of a professional healthcare provider if you are pregnant, nursing, or experiencing symptoms of any potentially serious condition.

# CONTENTS

# EXPANDED CONTENTS

# ACKNOWLEDGMENTS

THE WRITING OF THIS BOOK WOULD NOT BE POSSIBLE IF IT weren't for the invaluable and enormous contributions from a whole host of wonderful people. I want to extend my heartfelt gratitude to those people who have supported this work and me over a number of years. These people are, Rebecca Metro, Karen Bate, Nicola Dean, Dr. David Mickel, Dr. Derek Proudlove, Carol Clarke, Peter Haines, Clare Potter, Darryl Williams, Dr. Francis Teeney, Professor Roddy Cowie, Grete Bratberg, Leslee Beckvonpeccoz, Janelle Collard, Alison Lenihan, Maria Whiteley, Steve Rother, John Strydom, Jen Millward, and Paul Hawkins. In different ways these people have had a significant impact on the paths my work and life have taken.

A big thank you goes to all the clients that have chosen to work with me and trust me on their journey back to health. These are the individuals that have played such an enormous role in making this book possible.

I would like to thank Deborah Malmud, Kevin Olsen, Elizabeth Baird, Mariah Eppes, Natasha Senn, Julia Gardiner and everyone at W.W. Norton & Co for giving me the opportunity to write this book and for their on-going patience, guidance, and support.

A special thank-you to Dr. Gabor Maté for his foreword. When I was introduced to Gabor's work I was thrilled to see someone else boldly talking about the connection between stress, emotions and disease. His work continues to be an inspiration to me and many others.

Most of all I would like to thank my family for their love and support, particularly my wife Judith, daughters Isabel and Kimberly and my mother Hilary. When I was at school, my intention had been to pursue a career in sound engineering, but chronic tinnitus and the onset of a hearing impairment through the condition otosclerosis, had me rethink that. When looking at what to pursue at university my mother said, "why don't you think about psychology, you're good with people, everyone seems to come to you with their problems." That was probably the start of it…

# FOREWORD

KYLE DAVIES SET HIMSELF NO MODEST TASK IN WRITING *The Intelligent Body*. "The purpose of this book," he asserts, "is to guide you back to your true self." As many readers will find, if they apply his reasoning and guidance, the goal is achievable.

Davies approaches his subject with the simple intuitive awareness—arising from his clinical observations and amply documented by modern research—that mind and body cannot be separated. It follows that emotions help shape physiology. The suppression of emotions or their overindulgent expression may interfere with the healthy physiology of the human organism.

His clients come to him with constellations of symptoms: some non-specific such as headaches or anxiety, others classifiable under various diagnoses such as chronic fatigue syndrome, irritable bowel syndrome, fibromyalgia, or more medically "respectable" illnesses such as multiple sclerosis. Common to them all is stress the clients themselves have not acknowledged, life histories that have entrained emotional patterns that bespeak separation from gut feelings, identities based on external factors rather than a true valuation of the self, and difficulties regulating or, all too often, even fully experiencing, one's emotions.

His conclusions are startlingly similar to ones I arrived at as a physician and, again, completely in line with what modern science—tragically ignored in medical teaching and practice—has confirmed. First, for the most part, chronic illness is neither a random misfortune nor a genetically determined phenomenon, but an outcome of self-denying emotional patterns people unconsciously follow due to early conditioning. Second, these patterns wreak havoc with the body's physiology and express themselves in multiple forms, from vague symptoms to established disease. Third, and best of all, recognition and reversal of these patterns can alleviate symptoms, sometimes rapidly and dramatically, and in many cases can lead to the remission and even healing of disease.

As Davies expresses it, "there is a complex connection between your deep unconscious beliefs, your environment, and your behavior. The extent to which you are free to be who you really are, to experience and express yourself unleashed and unbridled and without the insidious shackles of past conditioning, can have a massive impact on your biology, neurology, physiology, and psychology." A massively positive impact, as he instructs and demonstrates in this volume.

The book is, in part, a compendium of research information. In part, it is a narrative of Davies' own education in the mind-body reality. It has been an education that, as in my own case and that of many other clinicians, has had to transcend and, often, consign to irrelevance, much of what is taught in the narrow confines of academic training. Davies had to unlearn to learn, as he urges his clients to do. And his best teachers, along with his own keen ability to observe, are his clients. Thus, for the most part, *The Intelligent Body* is not a theoretical work, but functions as the guide Davies set out to write.

And how do we get back to ourselves? Davies teaches many techniques to promote self-awareness, but he astutely warns that techniques are not the point: tapping into one's intuition is. He cautions the reader that, rather than a set of exercises to be followed mechanically, what he offers is "more like a body of knowledge that you need to understand and integrate." The exercises, he says, "are just designed to nudge you along the path to greater understanding and alignment with your true self. This book is offering you a perspective on how you work, how you function as a human being."

One of the first steps Davies recommends is letting go of any firmly held sense of identity, substituting instead a healthy curiosity about who we might really be. The principle is that a rigidly entrenched view of ourselves, conditioned by externally derived factors such as parental and social expectations, will interfere and block the natural experience of our innate drives and needs. Such blockages manifest in ill health; their release promotes healing.

Healing, ultimately, is the purpose of this book. And healing— rather than cure—resides in the inner capacities of body and psyche. It is promoted by agency, that is, the consciously self-directed capacity in each of us to guide our path according to our true nature. In what Davies rightly calls our "thinking and mind-centered society" we may not even realize we have a true nature, let alone be connected to it with full awareness. The epidemic of chronic illness in the industrialized world is as much the result of what we can call our *denaturation* as of any other factor, be it external stress, unhealthy diets, and sedentary lives. It is also the most insidious factor, the least likely to be identified by either the sufferer or his/her health practitioner.

*The Intelligent Body* is a welcome addition to the growing body of work intended to restore human beings to their true selves, to wholeness, to health. Davies' clinical successes have given him the confidence that such restoration, with health-enhancing benefits, is possible. In this book he lays out a path that, if diligently followed, will enable many to confirm through their own experience that similar successes can be attained in their own lives as well.

**Gabor Maté, MD**
Author, *When The Body Says No:*
*Exploring The Stress-Disease Connection*

# THE INTELLIGENT BODY

# PART I

## Building the Foundations

# CHAPTER 1

# Introduction

THE BUS GRINDS TO A HALT IN RURAL NEW HAMPSHIRE
and a group of elderly men shuffle off, their gaits heavily laden,
many afflicted with arthritis, hearing, and sight problems, and other
seemingly unavoidable health burdens that debilitate as age continues its relentless march. As they step cautiously through the door of
a converted monastery they are warped back in time twenty years,
to 1959. The black and white TV blinks and flickers as Jimmy Stew-
art plays the lead in *Anatomy of a Murder*, while the radio set churns
out another popular Perry Como classic. To the untrained observer
it would seem that we have literally stepped back in time; the books,
magazines, and decoration all paint a detailed picture of 1959. The
challenge facing these elderly men is to live as if it is 1959, to immerse
themselves completely and fully into their younger selves.

It was the Fall of 1979 and these men were taking part in a rad-
ical experiment that was the brainchild of Harvard Professor Ellen
Langer. The men would spend the week watching films, having dis-
cussions, and listening to radio shows while surrounded by props that
recreated the lives they had experienced as younger men. Langer was
interested in the impact this might have, not just on their outlook and
attitude but also their physiology. The men were all coddled to a certain extent by caring families who treated them as if they were old,
infirm, and incapable. Langer wanted to see what would happen to
them if this was reversed, so she started the week by inviting them to
carry their own suitcases from the bus to their rooms. The results of
her experiment were nothing short of remarkable. By the end of the
week the men displayed greater confidence and walked with more
ease and grace. But more interestingly, the physiological measure-

ments that Langer had taken all changed; gait, dexterity, arthritis, speed of movement, cognitive abilities, and memory all improved. Blood pressure dropped and eyesight and hearing difficulties were ameliorated.

The big question that arises from these incredible results is what caused them, how could these men's bodies literally change simply by immersing them in an environment they had encountered twenty years prior. It would be easy to assume this was mind over matter; positive thinking changes the body, it's all down to mindset. But that isn't the case. Conscious thought can't simply change your reality, otherwise I'm assuming you wouldn't be sitting reading this book—you'd be living your dream life in a paradise somewhere. There must be something deeper going on, something more that needs to be understood and investigated. Positive thinking isn't what is going to change your life, and was not the critical factor for the participants of Langer's experiment. However, there is a complex connection between your deep unconscious beliefs, your environment, and your behavior. The extent to which you are free to be who you really are, to experience and express yourself unleashed and unbridled and without the insidious shackles of past conditioning, can have a massive impact on your biology, neurology, physiology, and psychology. But what does it mean to be free, to experience all of who you can be, and how does this impact your health?

Whether we like to admit it or not, there is a deep connection between our health and vitality, our happiness, and our sense of fulfillment. The connection forms the premise of this book, and at its core it is remarkably simple. Optimum health, peace of mind, and a fulfilling life experience emerge when we are aligned with our "true self." You could call this your authentic self, your core, your inner wisdom, your internal guidance, your home base, your soul, your connection to source or higher consciousness; for our purposes it doesn't really matter. What is important is for us to know that there is a flow of consciousness that is *us*; it's more than our mind, in fact it's more than our physical body, but it is something that we can feel, something that we can sense, and something that we know. When we are aligned we feel good, life flows with ease, we have clarity and insight, and good experiences find their way to us. However, there are many things that get in the way, blocking us from aligning with our true self, and the more we deviate from this the more we feel lost, confused, and experience symptoms of health conditions such as chronic fatigue, pain, anxiety, and depression.

The purpose of this book is to guide you back to your true self. You don't achieve this through thought or rational analysis; you achieve this by allowing and flowing. Your true self is there within you waiting to be uncovered, to be unleashed. You know when you are aligned with it because you feel good, you flow. Realigning with your true self can happen in a moment or take a lifetime, all depending on what you do.

In the chapters to come, I will uncover the layers that make up this work, and explain how and why we become misaligned or disconnected and more crucially how to remedy the issue. The process can be like piecing together a puzzle; some parts will be particularly relevant and require attention, while others may not be as relevant to your particular situation and life circumstances. At times we will go deep into your relationship with yourself, and at other times the material may seem more like common sense. That said, let this book be your guide, let it facilitate your realignment with all of who you can be so that you can experience the very best of health, and the very best of yourself.

If you do suffer from a chronic health condition, this book is not meant as a replacement for appropriate healthcare advice and guidance, rather its purpose is to illuminate the path, to show you a new way and to give you a new understanding, and empower you to move towards health, vitality, and a fulfilling life.

## Are We Witnessing a Health Crisis?

Why are we appearing to see growing numbers of people in the Western world, suffering from debilitating chronic symptoms that medicine is failing to resolve? What creates this internal mayhem that sees the body seemingly break down with symptoms of pain, fatigue, bowel irritation and inflammation, and cognitive impairment?

Significant advances over the last half-century have seen medication as the focus of conventional healthcare. However, medication for the most part masks symptoms, blocks receptor sites, stimulates or suppresses the immune system, and ultimately only serves to ameliorate the symptoms without addressing their cause. This approach also leaves us very passive in the process of our own healthcare.

Treating symptoms doesn't deal with why the symptoms are present; it doesn't address the cause. The result can be that they will either persist or be replaced with another set of symptoms—almost as if our body is saying that if it can't get our attention with one set of symptoms, it will seek to grab our attention with another set. A new paradigm is needed, a paradigm where we understand the mind and body as an interconnected flowing system, connected to its environment, constantly changing and evolving, like a flowing stream. This paradigm embraces empowerment and understands the self-healing, self-correcting, and self-creating natures of our connected mind-body system.

Physical symptoms are simply a sign of disharmony and energetic imbalance, a "tap on the shoulder" from a body that is trying to get our attention. This "tap" on the shoulder can become a kick in the head, if we keep ignoring it. But when we pay attention, and understand this communication, we can take the steps to facilitate our own self-healing through an empowered process.

So, how can we possibly address and begin to reverse these seemingly chronic disorders? For those conditions where structural damage is present in the body, medical intervention is required (for example where tumors are present or in cardiovascular disease where heart muscle damage is evident). However, for those symptoms and syndromes where no structural damage is evident, health and vitality can be achieved through understanding the significant causes of symptoms and taking steps to address those causes. Even when structural damage is present future prevention and "damage limitation" is essential, and this is where the knowledge and understanding become paramount.

A new paradigm for healing is needed that has its roots in self-empowerment and vibrational change, addressing the cause and creating an environment within the body for health and wellness. As humans, we have an incredible capacity to heal ourselves. Most conventional healing modalities simply create an environment that allows the body to heal. If we break a leg, the common medical practice is to place a cast on the leg to protect it while the self-healing process takes place. However, we are also becoming more aware of the incredible power of the placebo effect, which suggests that healing can often take place simply through the belief that helpful medical intervention has taken place. Unconscious belief is difficult to control, but awareness, intention, and attention can be directed and utilized to good effect.

From a scientific perspective, it is "stressors" that prevent the body from healing itself. There is now a huge body of mainstream academic literature that supports the idea that the causes and maintainers of disease states is a body in a state of "stress." I do need to be clear that this form of stress is not nervous agitation, as we think of it in popular culture. Stress can't be defined merely as an internal feeling, because both animals and humans can be in a state of stress, without any awareness of its presence. Stress is a series of measurable physiological episodes inside the body. It is a biological alteration resulting from the interplay of emotion, cognition, our physiology, and external events and surroundings.

One of the early pioneers of the effects of stress on the body and its functioning was Dr. Hans Selye, and his theory known as General Adaptation Syndrome (GAS). In 1926, Selye defined stress as "the non-specific response of the body to any demand placed upon it." Despite the rather nebulous nature of this definition, it sufficiently represents the idea that an imbalance is present, and that it is this prolonged imbalance that will lead to the breaking down of body's systems, if left unresolved. Stress can result from physical injury, infection, trauma, or a perceived trauma, and all of these can affect biological functioning, as well as behavioral patterns and perceptions.

So, in other words, when a person's body is in a continued state of stress, it leads to disharmony and dissonance within the systems of the body, which leads to disruptions in the way the body functions. When there is disruption and the flow is affected, things start to break down. This is when we witness the manifestation of physical and psychological symptoms. It is only when internal and external balance is attained that the body can heal itself. The first step is for us to take a close look at what stress means and how it affects our body and brain.

CHAPTER 2

# It's Not the Stress You Feel, It's the Stress You Don't

*"No-one can live without experiencing some type of stress all
the time. You may think that only serious disease or intensive
physical or mental injury can cause stress. This is false.
Crossing a busy intersection, exposure to a draft, or even sheer
joy are enough to activate the body's stress mechanism to some
extent. . . . The same stress which makes one person sick can be
an invigorating experience for another."*

—Dr. Hans Seyle

I T WAS JUST AFTER 7:30, ON WHAT WAS A PRETTY REGULAR
morning. I'd done my usual routine in the shower of washing
everything in exactly the same order, getting out and drying. As I
started to fumble with my tie knot my attention was drawn by a piece
on the BBC-TV morning news. The presenter was telling me that academics had found a link between anger and heart disease. Anger and
heart disease in men—how on earth could that be the case? Anger is
an emotion. Emotions are all in the head, in effect, they are imaginary. How on earth could anger be linked to the real physical problem of heart disease?

A few months later, there was another piece on the very same
breakfast television BBC program. This time the presenter was telling me that there was a link between anger and heart disease in
women. So even though we generally think of men as having "anger
problems," getting all riled up, being destructive and aggressive, we
were now being told that women, whose displays of rage seem far

less frequent and explosive than men's, are also experiencing heart disease because of anger. Wow, my mind was blown; national television was going against everything that Western medical practice would teach us. But what did it mean, exactly? How could anger lead to heart disease, and what sort of an impact what this going to have on our healthcare system?

This information is revolutionary, when we think about the implications of it. If anger can somehow cause heart disease that means anger, and therefore all emotions, must actually be more than the "all-in the-mind" notion we have been led to believe. "It's not clear what causes this effect. It may be linked to the physiological changes that anger causes to our bodies, but more research is needed to explore the biology behind this," said Doireann Maddock, Senior Cardiac Nurse at the British Heart Foundation (BHF). Okay, so more research is needed. But more importantly mainstream science is now open to the idea that stress and disease are intimately connected.

Six months after this monumental revelation, I found myself reading an article in *The Observer* newspaper, a highly regarded London broadsheet. While sipping my steaming hot mug of black coffee, I came across a piece entitled, "Cancer Warning For Stressed-Out Men" I put my coffee down on the table and stared intently at the page. "Prostate cancer kills one man in Britain every hour and 10,000 each year—the equivalent of a Lockerbie air disaster every week." Professor Roger Kirby, chair of Prostate Cancer UK, a cancer research charity, said that many of these cases could be related to intolerable stress at work.

"We have to get men to look more to their feminine side," said Kirby, who is also editor of the journal *Prostate Cancer and Prostatic Diseases* and founder of The Prostate Centre in London. "They need to think and act more like women; share their emotions and focus on home and family, and less on pure career success. The changes that induce cells to become cancerous are unknown, but lifestyle is critical and men are creating the lifestyles that are killing them," said Kirby. I was certainly cognizant that research in the area was scant, and there would be those who would suggest that the views expressed by Professor Kirby were a little controversial. However, lack of sufficient data doesn't mean something isn't potentially true, it just means no one has bothered to research it yet, and there must be reasons for that.

This article transfixed me. It was 2007 and I had been working with sufferers of chronic health challenges for more than five years and it had felt like a complete uphill battle trying to get some recognition that mind and body were linked, that stress, emotion, and health were intimately connected. I was constantly told by people that the work I was doing couldn't be relevant because the conditions I worked with were "real" physical conditions, not psychological problems.

While the notion put forward by Professor Kirby that men should be more like women seems reasonable at one level, it struck me as being so oversimplified that it might damage the profound suggestion that stress could cause cancer. Uncovering data that might suggest that stress could cause cancer would most likely be the outcome of a highly complex and sophisticated process. Ideally what follows is a solution that is equally as rigorous and comprehensive. The solution wouldn't need to be complex; however, the suggestions of sharing emotions and focusing on home and family are too vague and woolly. First we need to understand stress and emotions and how they connect to health and disease.

## The Origins of Stress

*"Stress in heath and disease is medically, sociologically, and philosophically the most meaningful subject for humanity that I can think of."*

—Dr. Hans Selye

The origins of the word "stress" lie in the Latin word "strictus," meaning tightness, compression, or a narrowness. Yet we have to come all the way into the 18th and 19th centuries before the word "stress" enters everyday vernacular, where in industrial engineering the word was used to mean an abstract physical force, a pressure, or to put emphasis on something. In these contexts, the word stress was frequently used in conjunction or in collaboration with the word strain—stress being what was applied, and strain meaning what was felt or experienced.

The word stress has found permanent residence in today's parlance, but what does it actually mean, in the way we use it? The Oxford English Dictionary defines stress as: "Pressure or tension exerted on a material object." Or, in something a little more aligned to our current investigation: "a state of mental or emotional strain or tension resulting from adverse or demanding circumstances." If we turn our attention to a more healthcare-related definition, an online medical dictionary defined stress as: "an organism's total response to environmental demands or pressures."

One recurrent disagreement among researchers concerns the definition of stress in humans. Is it primarily an external response that can be measured by changes in glandular secretions, skin reactions, and other physical functions; or is it an internal interpretation of, or reaction to, a stressor; or is it both?

The term "stress" was originally used in the context of human experience by physiologist Dr. Hans Selye in 1926 to represent the interaction of the human body and the environment. Selye was born in Hungary in 1907, and came from a long line of physicians. He attended the German Medical School at age 17, and went on to attain a doctorate in organic chemistry. As a medical student, Selye learned that the primary focus in medical research was identifying specific markers for disease; this essentially means looking for measurable indicators of the presence and severity of a disease. Indicators would be identified and specific treatments and therapies would be developed or applied for specific diseases. Despite this system seeming like a perfectly sensible and logical approach to medical research, Selye was intrigued by patients who presented with symptoms and looked sick, without the specific markers. These patients would exhibit similar symptoms despite apparently having different conditions. Selye was fascinated by these "nonspecific" symptoms, and developed an interest in what were then called "nonspecific therapies"—meaning therapies that seemed to benefit a variety of health conditions. This was not a popular field of endeavor, and Selye faced significant resistance from his mentors and supervisors who suggested that pursuing this research interest would prove both futile and potentially career damaging. However, Selye's mind was made up and in 1936 he submitted a paper to the journal *Nature* outlining his theory on the nonspecific response of the body to demands placed upon it, which he called General Adaptation Syndrome (GAS). There are three phases of GAS: Activation, Resistance, and Exhaustion.

PHASE 1: ACTIVATION. This is where the body identifies or perceives a threat or stressor within the environment, and moves into the so-called "fight-or-flight" response—this is the body trying to retain homeostasis or balance by calling on the hormonal system. The first person to really examine the ability of the body to maintain constancy despite environmental changes and shifts was Claude Bernard, who delineated this in the 19th century. However, it was physiologist Walter Cannon who first coined the term *homeostasis* to describe the ability of the body to strive for balance, almost like the thermostat of your home's central heating system.

Homeostasis is also what is responsible for healing, or self-healing. When a schoolboy falls over and grazes his knee, there is nothing he needs to do in order for his knee to effectively heal. The natural mechanism of self-correcting homeostasis will endeavor to return the body to its original blueprint, or template. The only thing that can prevent a return to a healthy, graze-free knee would be perpetual falls onto the same knee, picking at the "scab," or some other process or mechanism that interrupts the body's natural flow and its self-healing system. Selye considered disease states to be the body fighting to maintain homeostatic balance; "Disease is not mere surrender to attack but also the fight for health; unless there is a fight, there is no disease."

During phase 1, fight or flight, the stress hormones cortisol, adrenaline, and noradrenaline are released and move throughout the body and brain. Increases in heart rate are evident, blood pressure will rise, and the activity within the emotional processing centers of the brain will become activated.

PHASE 2: RESISTANCE. Following the initial activation phase, the body remains in a state of arousal and continues to adapt to the existence of the stressor. In this phase the body is "coping" and working hard to maintain homeostasis. One of the significant differences between phase 1 and 2 is the level of awareness of the individual to the happenings within the body. Selye argued that in phase 2 the individual might be completely oblivious to the fact that the body is in adaptation mode with the stress response locked on. This of course is what makes this phase particularly dangerous. The body is in a state of stress, fighting to maintain homeostasis, but if this resides outside the conscious awareness of the individual nothing will be done to change the circumstances or interaction with the environment. The body can remain in this resistance phase for some time but not indefinitely. When the body's reserves have been depleted and can no longer maintain the "fight," phase 3 begins.

PHASE 3: EXHAUSTION. During this final phase the body's reserves are completely depleted and it loses its ability to maintain homeostasis and reduce the impact of the perceived stressors. Burnout sets in, and body systems begin to break down, as symptoms of illness and disease begin to present themselves. Selye was interested in the idea of "adaptation energy," and more specifically that we only have a finite amount of it available to us, as we seek to navigate through changing and challenging life circumstances. Selye believed that depletion of this adaptation energy arises from faulty adjustment to the environment, and it is the struggle to adjust to a changing or unfavorable environment that is responsible for many chronic diseases that are apparent in Western societies. Selye's conclusion was that stress plays a role in the causation of all disease, except those due to injury or infection.

The problem with Selye's concept of stress and its impact on the body lies in obtaining repeated consistent measurements. As stress is a nonspecific response of the body in its interaction with the environment, the response can vary between individuals and also can vary within an individual. So sitting in a draft may trigger a measurable response within the body one day and the following week a different response could be observed. This measured response could also be trigged by a variety of different environmental contexts. So despite pioneering this groundbreaking work on stress, many questions remained unanswered, and arguments continue within medical and academic circles.

## But What Does This Mean for Us?

The important understanding that arises from Selye's work is that stress is much more than the overwhelming agitated body discomfort that we can experience on a daily or weekly basis. Our body can be in a state of stress - adapting in phase 2 (Resistance), without us even being aware of it. That is the crucial issue. We are no longer living in the jungle being chased by tigers where the danger is pronounced and short lived. Modern life offers an entirely different breed of "threat." What we experience is a whole range of low-level "stressors" that keep us locked in the stress response without being aware of it. And, let's remember that we are going to look at stress as a symptom of our ability to adapt to our environment, that is our ability to be flexible in a number of ways. We are adaptable and flexible by nature. However, the irony is that the more stressed we become, the less adaptable and flexible we want to be, the more resistant we become.

The perspective presented in this book is slightly different from conventional views that seek to list external events that cause stress. We're used to seeing lists of disastrous occurrences such as job loss, relationship breakdown, moving house, etc., as being the most familiar causes of stress. However, it is not the events themselves that cause stress, rather it is our level of adaptability to those events. We cannot control external events and we do not need to. Life is life and we need to flow and move with it rather than trying to control it. I'm not suggesting that we are not affected by external events because we clearly are; however, our body responses are not fixed, they tend to vary. So the feeling response that arises from a certain set of circumstances one day may be different from that to the exact same set of circumstances the following day or week. From a young age, we tend to assume that external events directly cause and control how we feel. What emerges from this unconscious belief is a desire to control these external events. We could look at this as something of a spectrum, where at one end we have the idea that our feelings are directly linked to external events, and that a particular event will then lead to a particular feeling. At the other end of the spectrum, we have the idea that all emotions and feelings come from inside us, and are not influenced or related to external events. In my view, neither of these polar opposites is quite right. There is a sweet spot somewhere in the midpoint of this spectrum, where we recognize that our emotional feelings arise from inside us, while at the same time recognizing that we cannot extricate ourselves from our environment, that we are connected to the world around us. The purpose of this view is that when looking to understand our feelings we need to bring our attention back into ourselves rather than trying to manipulate external events. We'll talk more about this in the next chapter on emotion, but for now, let's return to the topic of stress.

## Stress, the Brain, and the Body

Advances in stress research have surpassed some of the original ideas of Selye, however his work was groundbreaking, and is absolutely vital in understanding the way that our body seeks to adapt internally to external changes. Stress is a hard-wired physical response, a set of objective measurable biochemical events that takes place through your entire body and brain, and is part and parcel of every day life. Stress is a reflection of the nature of our interaction with our environment. The stress response begins in the brain and body with the hypothalamic-pituitary-adrenal (HPA) axis. This is a collaboration between the endocrine glands in the brain and the adrenal glands that sit on top of the kidneys. When there is a perception of threat, the HPA axis is immediately activated. Short-term stress, which can trigger the fight-or-flight response in the body, is not problematic and does not negatively impact the body and brain. However, when the body remains in a state of stress, the adrenal glands release the stress hormones cortisol, epinephrine (adrenaline), and norepinephrine. These stress hormones course through your veins, affecting your blood vessels en route to your heart. Your heart will begin to beat faster and your blood pressure will rise. In the short term this "fight or flight" mobilizes you for action, preparing you to deal with a perceived threat. (Of course in the absence of an actual threat there is little need for these biochemical changes within the body.)

Over time if the stress response remains switched on these chemical changes can cause structural damage. Cortisol can lead to changes in the endothelium, where changes occur within the lining of the blood vessels. This can lead to atherosclerosis, where the lining of the arteries become clogged with plaque, or atheroma. Scientists believe that these changes can increase your chances of experiencing a heart attack or stroke. Chronic stress increases the neural connections within the amygdala, the brain's fear center, and leads to a deterioration of the electrical signals and a reduction in the number of new cells created within the hippocampus, the area of the brain involved in learning and the creation of new memories. This inhibits activity of the HPA axis, which weakens your ability to control or respond to stress. Too much cortisol results in the loss of synaptic connections between neurons and a shrinking of the prefrontal cortex—the executive center of the brain. This negatively affects concentration, decision-making, judgments, and social interaction.

The stress response can cause a chain reaction affecting the immune system, the endocrine system, and the autonomic nervous system (ANS). Through the ANS, there is a direct connection with the gut or digestive system. The trillions of bacteria that live in the body are called the microbiome and the majority of these reside in the gut—commonly referred to as the gut microbiota. The gut microbiota has its own neural network, the enteric nervous system (ENS), which scientists call the little brain. The ENS comprises two thin layers of more than a hundred million nerve cells lining your gastrointestinal tract, from esophagus to rectum. Modulation via the ANS can cause physical changes within the gut and your ENS. You'll be very familiar with the feelings of butterflies in the stomach. This is the mild impact of stress hormones impacting the stomach via the ENS. However, over time, chronic stress leads to irregularities within the stomach and digestive system which can manifest as symptoms of irritable bowel syndrome (IBS). The changes within the stomach leave it more sensitive to acid, which can result in heartburn or acid reflux. So stress can directly modulate or change the composition and nature of your gut bacteria and gut microbiota, which can have a massive impact on your health, through the immune system.

Stress hormones affect immune cells in a variety of ways, initially to fight infection or invaders and to facilitate healing. However, in the longer term with chronic stress, our body releases what are called inflammatory cytokines, little chemical messengers that bring a certain part of our immune system into high alert. In a sense, our body reacts to all stress as if it were an infection, and to chronic stress as if it were a chronic infection. The immune system does a great job with short-term inflammation to fight off pathogens like colds and flus; however, long-term inflammation is increasingly singled out as the primary contributor to a whole host of chronic health conditions, from depressive disorders to cancer.

## The Biomedical Model

For the last two hundred years, science has been dominated by a worldview assumption or doctrine of materialism, the idea that everything in the known universe is made of matter. The materialistic philosophy suggests that the universe is an enormous random machine, purposeless and directionless. Consciousness is seen as a byproduct of brain functioning, something that arises as a result of the biochemical and electrical activity that takes place between our ears. As human beings, we are, as the famous evolutionary biologist Richard Dawkins would say, "lumbering robots," playing out our genetic heritage, with no free will or choice.

We can't argue that science has seduced us all, and rightly so in many instances. We have seen almost miraculous transformations to the quality of people's lives through science, technology, engineering, and medicine. There has been something of an explosion of knowledge and our education systems have been focused on cascading this knowledge. The practical applications tend to focus on reductionism, which essentially means that in order to fully understand or explain something we need to break it down into its constituent parts. By breaking it down we will understand it, and this notion of reductionism often goes hand in hand with a linear mode of thinking.

When scientific materialism is applied to health, what emerges is the biomedical model. As with all scientific materialism, the biomedical model views the human body as a machine, random and purposeless, rather than as conscious people with their own subjective experience living in an environment, a system that is connected.

The modern-day foundations of the biomedical model could be traced all the way back to Girolamo Fracastoro, an Italian physician, poet, and scholar. At the age of 19, he was appointed as the professor at the University in Venice and in 1546 he made the bold claim that epidemic diseases are caused by transferable tiny particles or "spores" that could spread infection by direct or indirect contact, or even without contact over long distances.

Three hundred years later, Robert Koch and Louis Pasteur discovered that many infectious diseases were caused by the presence of microorganisms, which are microscopic, living, single-celled organisms, such as bacteria. Like most new ideas, Pasteur's discoveries were initially rejected, not least because he was a chemist and not a medical doctor. However, as acceptance to Pastor's work grew, it resulted in something of a paradigm shift in scientific understanding, overhauling the existing notion of health and disease that had been in existence since Aristotle. At the beginning of the 20th century, this theory—with its focus on the microorganisms that invade the human body, reproduce, and grow, ultimately causing chaos and leading to disease—was extremely successful in helping to dramatically diminish and eliminate diseases such as smallpox, tuberculosis, and influenza.

From Pasteur's work came the biomedical model of medicine. Conceptually, this model of disease suggests that illness is purely biological in orientation; psychological and social factors are excluded and not viewed as relevant aspects of the equation. The model has become the single approach used for the diagnosis and treatment of disease within mainstream healthcare in the Western world. The problem with the biomedical model is that it fails to explain many forms of illness, particularly many chronic illnesses that seem to be wreaking havoc in Western societies. Much like scientific materialism, the problem with the biomedical model lies in the underlying assumptions. These are that all illness has a single underlying cause, disease (pathology) is always the single cause, and removal or attenuation of the disease will result in a return to health.

## The Biopsychosocial Model

In 1977 psychiatrist George Engel questioned the linear and somewhat restricted biomedical model. He felt that the reductionist, analytical scientific medical approach was dehumanizing and disempowering patients. Engel believed that in order to effectively deal with patients' suffering, a more systemic and multi-leveled philosophy and approach was needed. Despite recognizing the significant advances within medical science, he was critical of the way that medicine was guiding clinicians to regard patients as objects largely ignoring their subjective experience. Engel felt that the individual could not be separated from the environment and that social and psychological factors need to be considered alongside biological ones. His ideology that health is impacted on a multitude of layers from the large-scale societal and cultural, through to the microscopic molecular, formed the basis of the biopsychosocial model.

Embracing this model when seeking to address chronic health challenges opens the door to a far greater range or possibilities for both cause and treatment. Moving away from a linear reductionist model of health and healing takes us towards a systems model and circular causality. This essentially means that if we are to look at the body as a complex system, biological, social, and psychological factors are all impacting each other—so everything affects everything else. This makes it very difficult to reduce things down to a single linear cause and opens up the possibility that there could be a combination of causes contributing to the onset of symptoms, almost like a combination lock—when all the numbers are aligned, the lock opens.

Obviously, we still need to be practical in the application of therapy or treatment, however, simply recognizing the systemic nature of the body and health, and being aware that contributory causal factors will emerge from biology, psychology, and the environment is important and valuable. What does this mean in practice? Critically it means that it is important to identify those aspects that relate to your health and that you can take charge of.

## Understanding the Stress Response

We've learned that stress is experienced when the body is working hard to maintain homeostasis, and we've also learned that the stress response calls into action all areas of the body and brain. Another interesting point is that the body's stress response is identical regardless of whether the stressor is a physical injury, an illness, or an emotional trauma. What this essentially means is that you could experience an illness, such as a case of flu, an emotional trauma, like having your car stolen, or have an accident or physical injury, such as falling down a flight of stairs, and the stress response that is triggered within the body is identical. When we combine the circular causality that we can take from the biopsychosocial model with Selye's GAS model, we could suggest that any combination of stressors could then trigger a disease state within the body. Let me explain this in more detail.

In working with clients with chronic fatigue, adrenal fatigue, and fibromyalgia, even anxiety and depression to a point, there is often, but not always, a single point in time that sufferers can pinpoint as being the start of their condition. Symptom onset is often traced back to a case of Epstein-Barr or infectious mononucleosis (IM), also known as glandular fever; several of my clients have reported car crashes as preceding the onset of symptoms; and in many instances emotional trauma such as job loss and bereavement. As we embrace the notion of circular causality and the combination lock of primary causes, we could argue that these identifiable causes are possibly the proverbial last straw that tipped the body's stress response into exhaustion.

For the purposes of simplicity, I like to use a "stress bucket" anal-ogy (see diagram below). Imagine for a moment that you have a bucket inside and every time your body's stress response is triggered the bucket fills up a little bit more. When the bucket is full and begins to overflow symptoms present themselves. The biggest contributors are blocked or unprocessed emotions, which can constantly drip into the stress bucket. Poor nutrition and excessive strenuous exercise are easier fixes because they are more obvious and tangible, and in my view, not as significant as a constant emotional blockage and imbal-ance. That's not to say that they are not significant because they are. However, as most things, even food and fitness, are connected to emotion in one way or another, it is usually the case that emotions exacerbate the impact on the body. I have worked with clients who have reported experiencing their symptom onset following a great deal of strenuous exercise and in all of these cases they were either walking around with a full stress bucket already or were using exer-cise as a means to overcome stress or to get away from emotional overwhelm. This puts a whole new slant on the idea of exercise being a great stress reliever. In instances where we are dealing with a rel-atively empty stress bucket this is true. However, in those instances

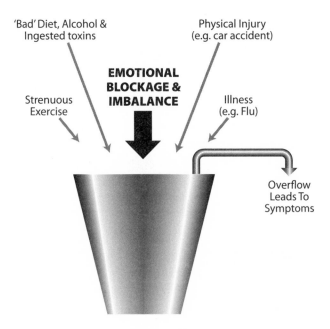

where the stress bucket is pretty full working out strenuously could have negative consequences, especially when exercise is an attempt to escape stress.

I certainly factor this into my life. I like to hit the gym pretty hard, but I am extremely aware of how my body feels and how full my stress bucket is. Have you ever had the experience of feeling a cough or cold coming, on and then you exercise strenuously? Sometimes the workout seems to do the trick and you feel better, while other times it seems to facilitate the onset of viral symptoms. If you've ever wondered why this is, a plausible argument is that your stress bucket is pretty full, and the combination of virus plus strenuous exercise was sufficient to weaken the body and allow the virus to take hold.

For our purposes in this book, the focus is on emotional blockage and imbalance—and we'll talk more about the true nature of emotion in the next chapter. If we were to map this out in a slightly different way, we could suggest that a prolonged buildup or imbalance of emotional energy leads to a rewiring of neural pathways within the emotional midbrain, which in turn leads to irregularities within the major systems of the body: the autonomic nervous system, the endocrine system, and the immune system. The end result of this dysfunction is the onset or presence of symptoms and disease.

If we allow ourselves to entertain this theory we can see why treating symptoms or trying to balance, boost, or work on the immune, endocrine, and nervous systems fails to effectively address probably the most significant of causes. Because of the circular nature of causality, addressing nutritional deficiencies via supplements and others means will support the body in the process of healing. However, if we fail to address the persistent suppression and blocking of emotion, recovery could be a challenge.

## Long-term stress path

| Long-term Emotional Imbalance (Stress) | Build up of Stress Hormones | Over-activity in Mid-Brain | Dysfunction in body systems | Symptoms and disease |
|---|---|---|---|---|

**Chain Reaction** →

You might be wondering why this idea about stress and disease is not having the impact on practices within mainstream healthcare. There are two answers to that question: First, we seem to be witnessing a gradual yet persistent academic tide tying together the impact of long-term stress on the body and the onset of symptoms and disease. Second, what continues to present itself is that sufferers of chronic health challenges such as chronic fatigue syndrome, fibromyalgia, and adrenal fatigue are often vociferous in their resistance to any theory and practice that entertains the idea of emotion or stress as a factor. This is because stress and emotion are still classed as "all in the mind" phenomena and not relevant to real physical diseases. Despite being antiquated and outdated, the notion of a separate mind and body is still the prevailing doctrine within mainstream medical practice.

If you are reading this and have been one of those people who have resisted any idea, notion, theory, or practice that is not firmly grounded in the physical and medical, now is your opportunity to recognize that stress is a complex physiological process that can result in body systems going haywire over a period of time.

## Mind-Body Dualism

This may be a bold statement, but I believe that intuitively people know there is a connection between how they feel and their health, their emotion, and their well-being. But standard medical practice still presupposes the mind-body split. The body is seen as a machine. If things go wrong with that machine the individual part is treated. The symptoms are treated. This dualistic view of mind and body is what prevents us from embracing the potential impact of stress and emotion on the functioning of our bodies. And what is most interesting is that even though the foundation is believed to be a desire to focus on hard measurable science, the notion of a mind-body separation or split originates in a worldview assumption.

With each generation there emerges a way to perceive the world and our role in it. A way of seeking to understand how everything fits together, why we are here, where we are going, what's it all about. The prevailing doctrine that has dominated our worldview assumption has been "Cartesian dualism." Dualism is an ancient concept, with both Plato and Aristotle reasoning that the human soul, psyche, or mind was different and separate from the physical body. René Descartes took this idea further and gave it the name "dualism." Descartes lived at a time when science was developing yet as religious men, the thinkers and scientists of the day needed to find some way of including God within their philosophical notions of the world. Man, being different from other animals and objects had a soul and this soul was not material. It was beyond the physical and represented man's connection to God. Descartes thought that the physical body could be separated into distinct parts, as in arms and legs that were machine-like, whereas the soul was different—it could not be split apart, separated, or measured. Scientists that have followed Descartes's philosophy have adapted this doctrine of the mind-body split and in an attempt to remove God from the equation the soul has been replaced with the mind. Thus emotions and feelings have taken the place of the psyche and the soul.

As we entertain the new perspective of the nature of stress and its role and impact on body and brain, we can see that the notion of a separate mind and body is outdated and no longer useful, and that in fact continuing to embrace it hinders progress. What is crucial for us as we seek to address and overcome chronic and debilitating health challenges, is to integrate the notion that mind and body are one. We cannot separate the individual from his environment and we cannot separate the mind from the body. As human beings we are one undulating, complex system of flowing interactions. Over the years I have come across many people who enthusiastically proclaim their agreement with a holistic philosophy that states the connection between mind and body, only to then talk about emotion and stress as concepts that are in the mind and not actually real or physical. As we have learned through the biomedical model, we need to recognize that an invading pathogen or germ can cause illness just as an accident can lead to broken bones or torn ligaments. While the cause of these is evident, the impact on the body is not necessarily significantly different from the impact on the body and brain caused by long-term stress or emotional overload.

So how do we embrace the mind-body connection? First, we accept that a physical symptom is simply a manifestation, and that this manifestation could be interpreted as feedback from a body that is locked in the stress response, even if we aren't consciously aware of it. Second, we have to take a look at our ideas about cause and effect. As humans, we naturally like to see cause and effect as being very closely linked together. An example is that if I have a stomachache it must be something that I have eaten, something I have put inside my stomach. The biomedical model has encouraged linear rather than systems thinking, which further encourages us to see cause and effect as being very closely linked together. However, the idea that symptoms of anxiety, depression, fatigue, or pain could be caused by an emotional stressor or even a nutritional deficiency pushes cause and effect further apart. When we contextualize that emotional stressor, it becomes even harder to see the connection.

Here's an example of a recent conversation with a client to exemplify the difficulty in reconciling the gap between cause and effect. My client said, "Are you saying that when my boss asks me if I can do a load of extra work, and even though it's pretty unfair, I agree to it, then later on I have an increase in symptoms of pain and fatigue, that these symptoms are related to that interaction with my boss?" and I say, "Yes, that's exactly right."

Why is this difficult? Because we have become inculcated into the biomedical model of thinking that presupposes that symptoms are signs of disease, and disease is either an infection or an accident. As we entertain a systems model and circular causality, we can open up our ideas about cause and effect and embrace the role of stress in health.

## What Role Does Trauma Play?

Trauma is a massive topic, with a multitude of books written on the subject all seeking to understand the impact that it has on health and how to recover. Like many stressors, it is the invisible cost, the hidden damage of trauma that we are only just beginning to really understand. There is currently a growing interest in the role that adverse childhood experiences, or ACEs, play in later life. It seems that emotional trauma and early life stress can have a profound impact on our biology over time and significantly increase the likelihood of experiencing chronic health challenges as we grow older.

ACEs are traumatic childhood events, ranging from emotional, physical, or sexual abuse, to family dysfunction and health challenges, and parental neglect or incarceration. While we often think about trauma in terms of hugely significant events, the drip feed of low-level emotional stressors in childhood can prove equally impactful over time. The origins of this work can be traced back to 1985 and the research of Dr. Vincent J. Felitti, chief of Kaiser Permanente's Department of Preventive Medicine in San Diego. At the time, Felitti ran an obesity clinic within the department and was somewhat frustrated and puzzled by a disturbing 50 percent dropout rate from his obesity program. What didn't seem to make sense to him was that those who were dropping out were losing weight, not gaining weight, meaning the program must have been working.

Felitti was eager to understand why the obesity program was apparently failing, so he dug deep into the medical records to understand the bigger picture of what was taking place. All of the participants were normal weight at birth, and had not gained weight gradually over time. Rather they seemed to gain weight abruptly and then stabilize. With this information, Felitti decided to interview a couple of hundred participants to see if he could glean any further insight. Almost by accident he uncovered that early life stress may play a role. When asking a subject about her weight and initial sexual experiences, it became apparent that she had been the victim of sexual abuse. Concerned by this finding, he invited colleagues to assist with further interviews. Of the 286 participants interviewed, almost all of them had been victims of sexual abuse. As these staggering results were sinking in, Felitti had the realization that the reason why so many were dropping out of the obesity program was because they didn't see their weight as a problem; eating was a fix, it was a solution. Like any other drug, or even self-harm, eating soothed the pain, and temporarily solved the problem. If they lost weight, they would experience a significant rise in fear, anxiety, depression, and anger. The potential implications of these early findings were mind-blowing.

The next step was a huge research study. As the largest medical evaluation site in the world, the preventative medical center screened more than 50,000 people every year, collecting data and screening for disease before symptoms appeared. Felitti put together a research team, which included additional trauma-oriented questions in their data collection methods. These questions focused on three types of abuse—physical, verbal, and sexual—and five types of family dys-function: an alcoholic or mentally ill parent, a parent suffering from domestic abuse, a family member who has been in prison, loss of a parent through divorce or abandonment, and emotional neglect. This gave ten distinct categories of ACE that could be used to inter-pret results when the data was collected.

Data was analyzed from more than 17,000 members of Kai-ser Permanente's San Diego care program, and what emerged was nothing short of staggering. Almost two-thirds of study participants reported at least one ACE, and more than one in five reported three or more ACEs. The more ACEs a child had experienced, the greater the chances of developing health and social problems later in life. Results revealed that ACEs could be linked to every major chronic illness and social problem evident in the USA. These included cancer, heart disease, stroke, chronic lung disease, multiple sclerosis, chronic fatigue syndrome, autoimmune conditions, chronic depression, and anxiety, and social and behavioral issues including substance abuse, time spent in prison, relationship difficulties, unintended pregnan-cies, suicide attempts, risk of sexual violence, poor academic achieve-ment, poor work performance and absenteeism—and this list is not exhaustive.

The notion that something that happened to you as a kid could end in hospitalization with a chronic health condition at age 50 is more than a little disturbing. The reason lies in the stress response and its implications over time. When the fight-or-flight response is frequently triggered it can impact the structure of the developing brain. Children in an environment of chronic toxic stress begin to interpret the world as a place of perpetual danger. This is not a con-scious decision, it's a direct result of how the brain structure adapts to the environment. When the brain and body are overloaded with stress hormones early in life the stage is set for problems later in life, as well as for difficulties in childhood.

The study uncovered how ACEs are risk factors for disease, and charted the relationship in a pyramid-type structure. At the base are the adverse childhood experiences that lead to disrupted neuro-development; this in turn leads to social, cognitive, and emotional impairment, leading to the adoption of health risk behaviors, such as drug and alcohol misuse, which in turn leads to disease, disabil-ity, and social problems, and ultimately early death. What was once thought of as an uncommon problem of early life stress and trauma is far more pervasive than anyone imagined.

And it doesn't end there. It would appear that the impact of trauma can begin to affect us even before birth. Professor Rachel Yehuda, at the Traumatic Stress Studies Division at the Mount Sinai Medical Center, in New York, conducted a longitudinal study with women who were pregnant and either in or near the World Trade Center on 9/11. The research showed that those who suffered from PTSD had lower cortisol levels, and this was somehow passed on to their offspring. The result of these lower cortisol levels in the children was a more rapid and significant distress response, when presented with something new or novel; their bodies and brains would get flooded with inflammation at even minor triggers. The pertinent question is therefore how were mothers passing on the impact of their trauma to their children.

The answer to this question is arguably addressed in research conducted by Dr. Joan Kaufman, director of the Child and Adolescent Research and Education (CARE) program, at the Yale School of Medicine. Kaufman and colleagues found that early life stress caused epigenetic changes that lowered the trigger required for a stress response. Epigenetic refers to the external modifications to the DNA that switches genes "on" or "off," and impacts how the cells of the body interpret and read genes. So it would seem that a pregnant mother enduring trauma will epigenetically effect her child, even before it is born.

What is evident here is that both significant trauma and a drip feed of low-level early life stressors could ultimately lead to significant negative consequences later in life. Early life stress can be triggered through chronic domestic disharmony and the prevalence of negative emotions accompanying a whole host of unpleasant life experiences. What is important is that we not only understand and learn from these studies but also that we seek to move towards finding solutions. Epigenetic changes are potentially long-lasting, but not necessarily permanent. The brain continues to develop and change as we grow. Stress and emotion arise as a result of the way we are interacting with our environment today, so it therefore must be possible to change our biology, physiology, neurology, and psychology by taking charge of stress, emotion, and ultimately ourselves, today.

## What Connects Stress and Medically Unexplained Symptoms?

In the UK, USA, and other Western nations, we are witnessing significant increases in what medicine refers to as medically unexplained symptoms. In the UK, over thirty percent of symptoms reported by patients presenting at primary care and over 50 percent of symptoms presented at secondary care are medically unexplained. This essentially means that medicine can find no biological reason for the presence of such symptoms. These symptoms and syndromes have been referred to as medically unexplained symptoms, functional symptoms, or functional somatic symptoms, and more recently as bodily distress disorders. This doesn't mean these symptoms don't exist, that they're not real, or that they are all in the mind. It simply means that the medical profession does not have a mechanism for identifying why these symptoms are present.

The most common functional symptoms are:

- Persistent headaches and migraines.
- Stomach and bowel problems including acid reflux.
- Persistent pain symptoms, including chest, neck, shoulder, and back pain (where there is no structural damage).
- Skin conditions including hives and psoriasis.
- Fatigue or weakness for more than just short periods of time.
- Insomnia.

When clusters of symptoms appear together, they are classed as syndromes. These are:

- Myalgic Encephalomyelitis (ME)
- Chronic Fatigue Syndrome (CFS)
- Post Viral Fatigue Syndrome (PVFS)
- Chronic Fatigue and Immune Dysfunction Syndrome (CFIDS)
- Fibromyalgia
- Irritable Bowel Syndrome (IBS)

What is important about these symptoms is, first, the primary cause will in a huge number of instances be related to stress and an overflowing stress bucket. Second, these symptoms are not causing structural damage or abnormalities to the body, so these symptoms can be reversed without invasive medical treatments that are so often adversarial and cause systemic damage to other areas of the body.

## Why Are We Seeing an Increase in These Symptoms and Conditions?

So, medically unexplained symptoms and syndromes are increasing, but why? Is it simply because of the way statistics are recorded? Are we allowing ourselves to wallow in health niggles, rather than just getting on with it? I suspect not. But I do think that it has something to do with the way we live our lives. Our modern society sees us continually rushing around in a semi-trancelike state, always on the go, always focusing on the next thing that has to be done. We can be like hamsters on a wheel with our busy consumer-driven lifestyles. The vast majority of us are stuck in a cycle of debt, feeling like wage slaves, living in an almost constant state of fear and concern. We worry about how we will pay our bills and afford to buy the things that we think we need. There is significant and constant pressure to conform, to be successful, to appear happy. Life seems to have become so complex that unless you have a great career, are well-traveled, are having almost daily amazing life experiences, and are constantly "up for it," there is something wrong. Clearly social media indoctrinates this life view, but the reality is somewhat different, in that most people are nowhere near experiencing this notion of an ideal life.

In truth, we have become lost. We have lost our connection to ourselves, to each other, to nature and the world around us, and to our sense of something greater than ourselves. The pressure of modern life has left significant collateral damage, as more and more people feel out of control, miserable, and hopeless, with failing health. When we experience emotional discomfort or ill health we are encouraged to take a pill or medication and get on with the day-to-day business of running around the hamster wheel. Our television screens are covered with adverts for products that merely bandage our symptoms—pills and patches for back pain, joint pain, and headaches, potions to help us sleep and to wake us up, and products to mask our acid reflux and help our bowel movements. All these "quick fix," superficial remedies have made us very passive in relation to healthcare, we seem to have been lulled into a disempowered state where we give responsibility for our health to someone or something else, and rarely address the underlying cause of symptoms.

## The Hallway of Health

Chronic health challenges such as CFS, fibromyalgia, adrenal fatigue, and related conditions don't appear out of the blue. There is a process by which symptoms appear and disappear. When I ask my clients to tell me their medical history and experience of symptoms, they initially tell me when they received a diagnosis—and in many instances this will have taken a frustratingly protracted period of time—then they often pause, think, and tell me about symptom episodes that trace back to childhood. These usually include unexplained stomach upset, headaches, inability to sleep, anxiety, and even a groggy fatigue.

The gradual increase in symptoms is something I call the Hallway of Health. Let's start by using hunger as an analogy; for the average person a mild rumbling sensation is a common occurrence to alert us to the fact that our body wants some food. Of course we can argue that we can train the body to be hungry at certain times by eating at the exact same time every day. However, that said, if we push that mild rumbling sensation to one side, it will tend to subside. Then at some point later, it returns, and when it returns, it tends to be a little more intense and it may be a little more uncomfortable. Rather than the nice pleasant rumbling, you're now experiencing something that is bordering on discomfort. If you continue to ignore this new "symptom," it may subside for a while, before returning again. If this were to go on for several days, the mild rumbling will be completely replaced by something more akin to significant discomfort. You might even feel faint, weak, and unable to function properly. The "symptoms," whether mild or severe are alleviated in exactly the same way, by ingesting the right amount of the right food for you.

Does the body work in the same way with other stress-related symptoms? Is there something of an ebb and flow where symptoms increase and decrease, appear and disappear? It is certainly the case that most people who experience acute symptoms, ranging from hangovers and headaches to symptoms of flu or back pain will be aware that symptoms can come and go in waves. However, there is something else going on when we look at how acute symptoms become chronic symptoms. There is still the pattern of ebb and flow as symptoms increase and decrease but this is coupled with an overall general increase in intensity and severity of symptoms.

As I collected the medical histories of clients, well-established patterns would reveal themselves. The onset of acute medically unexplained symptoms of fatigue, pain, or even anxiety and depression, we are going to call stage 1 of the Hallway of Health. Those initial symptoms, whether treated or not, very often subside either for a short period of time or for something a little longer term. When the symptoms return at stage 2 they tend to be more severe, more intense and in some instances to be different symptoms altogether. Finally there is stage 3 in our Hallway of Health. At this stage, sufferers would experience chronic fatigue syndrome, fibro, multiple sclerosis, and autoimmune conditions.

I remember several years ago talking with a client who was a family physician, a GP. She was suffering from multiple sclerosis and had been looking for some alternative ideas of how to address or even understand what she was experiencing. I told her about the anecdotal theory of the Hallway Of Health and she listened intently and then proceeded to tell me how quite recently she had taken a whole filing cabinet full of patient case notes and had seen a progression of illness. She told me that she could see how patients had come presenting minor symptoms, she would offer medication and then at some point later they would return with more severe symptoms. She said that in pretty much all instances where a patient was presenting with a chronic debilitating health challenge, she could see a pattern of symptoms gradually getting worse, interspersed with periods of relatively good health and vitality.

Let's take a close look at the three stages of the Hallway to Health as they appear.

STAGE 1: Headaches, stomach upset, insomnia, mild groggy fatigue, skins rashes, to moderate anxiety or depression, frequent coughs, and colds.

STAGE 2: Symptoms from Stage 1 begin to cluster or become more intense; for example, headaches coupled with some stomach aches and pains. Or anxiety coupled with groggy fatigue. Stage 2 is where signs of full-blown IBS presents itself and where autoimmune disease begins.

STAGE 3: This is where full-blown ME, CFS, post-viral fatigue, fibromyalgia, adrenal fatigue, chronic immunodeficiency syndrome, and multiple sclerosis present themselves. Stage 3 is also where mild to moderate anxiety or depression could become severe anxiety or depression. If we were to compare the symptoms of someone suffering from severe depression and someone suffering CFS, in many instances there would be a huge amount of overlap.

As you might expect, as this is a hallway it is possible to walk up and down it, and that is exactly what sufferers do. This is why it's possible to experience different symptoms at different times. I've had so many clients over the years that have reported a lessening of CFS symptoms, only to see an increase in anxiety symptoms or psoriasis which they hadn't experienced in 10 years. I formally congratulate them on their progress and they usually look at me as if I'm crazy. "It's okay" I say, "you're making progress, you're walking back down the Hallway to Health. You changed direction and rather than it being the Hallway From Health you're walking back down the Hallway To Health." [1]

## Where Do Anxiety and Depression Fit?

As you can now see, we are entertaining a mind-body model that does not make an absolute distinction between mental health and physical health. Yes we can experience mental or emotional symptoms and physical symptoms, but where the symptoms manifest may have nothing to do with the cause of those symptoms.

CFS sufferers often vociferously argue that they don't have depression, and I'm not suggesting that CFS and depression are the same thing. However, when we look at anxiety and depression, we can see that they are umbrella terms for a diverse range of psychological and physical symptoms, in much the same way as CFS and fibromyalgia are umbrella terms themselves. Depression is not simply low mood; sufferers can also experience fatigue, and even muscle aches and pains. The most important element for us to remember is that

---

1   (This progression was first noted by therapist, David Greenshields and further developed by my former colleague, Dr. David Mickel.)

we are viewing the significant primary cause as an overflowing stress bucket, which causes inflammation within body and brain, leading to a host of debilitating symptoms.

You may wonder why it is that one person exhibits symptoms of depression or anxiety, while another presents with symptoms of fatigue or stomach upset. While I don't have a definitive answer to that question, I suspect that it is our genetic lineage that plays the biggest role in what symptoms present themselves. We all hold the genetic potential or predisposition for a whole range of health challenges yet only a small proportion actually manifest into disease states. The new and growing field of epigenetics suggests that it is our interaction with the environment that has the greatest impact on whether these health challenges actually manifest.

## Beyond Food and Fitness

Without doubt we are experiencing a wave of change in the world of healthcare, with more people seeking to take charge of their own health and well-being. Regular exercise and optimal nutrition are important for a healthy life. They have implications for our bodies' stress response and our gene expression (epigenetics). However, current thinking and wellness trends seem to promise that food and fitness are a panacea for all ills. If you exercise and eat well, taking the right supplements, you'll feel good, be healthy, and free from any symptoms or health problems. Unfortunately, this is simply not the case.

The real scientific understanding of nutrition is still reasonably rudimentary, and this possibly explains why there are so many divergent and contrasting theories on what to eat and what to avoid. We've all heard the purported benefits of a vegetarian or vegan diet, while others promote the paleo model with plenty of grass-fed meat. With so many competing theories on what to eat and what to avoid, real scientific evidence seems to be either misinterpreted or lacking.

While there may be no "one-size-fits-all" model of nutrition, I believe too much emphasis is placed on food's potential ability to eradicate all symptoms of disease, elevate your mood, and leave you a happy, confident individual. To be clear, I'm not against exercise and nutrition, in fact I am a big fan. I love to exercise and I train at the gym three to four times a week. I am conscious of what I eat and how I cook. I am interested in the scientific research that underpins both these fields, and I follow the work of those who disseminate good research, ideas, and theories. I am conscious that both nutrition and exercise play a role in what goes in our stress bucket and therefore the level of inflammation in the body.

That said, when looking to achieve total wellness, I believe the most important piece of the puzzle is often missing: emotions. Exercise and nutrition are key pillars for health, but crucially it is the balance of physical, emotional, and spiritual that provides the underpinning foundation for health, happiness, and fulfillment. Understanding the mental, emotional, and spiritual aspects of life— everything from how we interface with life in every moment of every day, to the deep unconscious relationship we have with ourselves and our "soul"—is crucial to true wellness and fulfillment in life.

The point I am seeking to make in this chapter is that there is increasing acceptance that stress, through the process of adaptation within the body, will cause disease. The point of this book is not to go into great detail about the biophysiological mechanisms that lead to a modulation in the endocrine, nervous, and immune systems that ultimately lead to disease; rather we are taking as a given that stress will lead to health challenges. What we need to do is understand the relationship between stress and emotion, how they are different, and how we can use this knowledge to move towards better health and happiness.

# CHAPTER 3

# What's Feeling Got to Do with It?

*"We're not just little hunks of meat. We're vibrating like a
tuning fork—we send out a vibration to other people. We
broadcast and receive. Thus the emotions orchestrate the
interactions among all our organs and systems to control that."*

—Dr. Candace Pert

IT WAS DUSK AND THE RAIN WAS COMING DOWN IN SHEETS.
Driving conditions were increasingly difficult as visibility seemed
to diminish with each wall of rain that descended from the skies.
The radio churned out something forgettable, but was barely audible
under the drone of raindrops pounding the car. Out of the corner of
my eye I could see a blue Mazda, winding its way in and out of traffic,
slaloming and vying for position as the lines of cars worked their way
north. Car horns sang out above the banging rain as the Mazda raced
Formula 1–style, forgetting this was in fact the daily commute home
and there was no prize money and flowing Champagne waiting at
the finish line. As the Mazda came perilously close to me, swirling
around then darting in front almost taking a chunk of my car with
him, I could feel a surge of sensation course though my body. The
sensations seemed to start in my chest before radiating across the
back of my shoulders and down my arms. They were not particularly
significant, but as I allowed myself to observe them they sparkled all
over my body like fireflies in the night, setting everything momentarily alight. The urge to think or react presented itself, but I'd grown
wise to the dangers of allowing such folly to rampage my system and
overrun my deeper wisdom and true self's calling. I observed, curi-

ous as to where the sparkling sensations in my body would go, and where my true self would pull me.

These sensations that were moving so fluently throughout my body and brain were of course emotional feelings. But what are feelings and emotions? Are they imaginary, something that just takes place in your head, the end result of your thinking; do they help or hinder you; are emotions and feelings the same thing or are they in some way different? It seems to me that there are so many different ideas about what emotions and feelings are that confusion quickly arises. If you were to consider the question, "what is an emotion?" I'm sure, to begin with, you would reflect on your own life experience to see the role emotion has played for you, and of course your subjective experience is extremely valid. It is your truth. In our desire to quantify and measure everything about life, the objective hard scientific view is often seen as the benchmark of truth. So what can academics offer us, as we seek to understand and make sense of emotions and feelings? A brief look reveals that there are an array of different ideas as to what emotion means, and for the most part the different theories address the issue from a variety of perspectives—a bit like the old story of the blind men describing an elephant through touch, each one holding and touching a different part and offering a different description of what an elephant actually is based on their immediate sensory experience. However, what seems to be missing from the predominant theories of emotion is the role it plays in health and well-being—which is exactly our area of interest.

In this chapter we are going to learn that emotion is critical and fundamental to life. Without emotion we would do nothing. Emotion and the feelings associated with emotion drive everything both conscious and unconscious. Even when we think we are engaged in emotion-free rational thought, our emotion is playing a role, influencing, coloring, and directing the nature of our thinking and resulting behavior. As a complex physiological process, our emotion affects our body and brain in significant ways. Emotion plays a far greater role in the emergence and persistence of chronic pain and fatigue conditions than is currently thought.

## The Academic View

When I studied psychology at university, I don't think I saw the word "emotion" mentioned in any of the textbooks. Psychology in the 20th century was trying its best to be a bona fide "hard science," like physics, chemistry, and biology. In the 1920s to 1950s the prevailing paradigm in mainstream psychology was behaviorism with its focus on measuring behavior. The internal workings of the mind or psyche were disregarded in favor of the objective and observable. Behaviorism gave way to the cognitive revolution and the study of mental processes as interest in the brain and neuroscience grew. Somehow the serious study of emotion fell through the net. That's not to say emotion was completely ignored, but it didn't enjoy the same level of attention as other areas of psychology. In saying that there are now a number of theories and schools of thought pertaining to emotion within mainstream academia. Let's take a very brief look at the main ideas.

In modern Western science, Charles Darwin first wrote about emotion in the 1870s, where he compared the expression of emotion in animals to the expression in humans. Darwin was primarily interested in mapping evolution and finding "matches" for his theory. His work was aimed at understanding the connections and overlap between animal and human experience. When looking at emotion this is most obvious in facial expression; Darwin found that people of different cultures and from different countries all expressed emotion facially in much the same way. Emotions such as fear, anger, and sadness all had common facial expressions. Darwin went a stage further to suggest that there was a common set of emotions experienced by all species. These included, anger, fear, sadness, and surprise.

Following Darwin's work, the great American psychologist, William James, posed the question in his seminal paper titled, *What Is An Emotion?*, published in 1884. James was of the view that emotion originated in the body and was primarily a visceral experience. He suggested that emotions were no more than bodily changes experienced as a result of external stimuli. So if we were to confront a tiger in the jungle we would immediately run and the perception of running and the resulting bodily changes would give rise to the emotion of fear. This theory was supported by Danish physician, Carl Lange in the 1880s. The resulting James-Lange theory that emotions arise from physiological changes in the body was one of the earliest and most significant theories of emotion within modern psychology.

In the 1920s, neurologist Walter Cannon challenged the James-Lange theory. Cannon wasn't convinced by the theory that emotion was dependent on interpreting the body's physiological reaction.

He felt that more of a neurobiological explanation was needed, and argued that emotions originated in the brain rather than the body, as James had suggested. In an attempt to prove this, he performed experiments on monkeys where he directly stimulated their brains. Despite not being as profound or intense as regular emotional experience, Cannon observed that the monkeys experienced emotional sensations as a result. He argued that bodily changes were too slow to generate emotions, and that stimulating brain regions alone was sufficient to produce emotions.

This theory proposed by Cannon was later developed by his doctoral student, Phillip Bard. What emerged was the Cannon-Bard theory, which states that we feel emotions and experience physiological reactions such as sweating, trembling and muscle tension simultaneously, so an external stimulus triggers both arousal and emotion at the same time. For example, hearing breaking glass might lead to an increase in your heart rate and a dilation of your pupils at the same time as the subjective experience of fear.

Drawing on both the James-Lange, and Cannon-Bard approaches, were Stanley Schacter and Jerome Singer, in 1962. Their "two-factor" model of emotion ushered in a cognitive approach and stated that some external stimulus (our "broken window") leads to internal arousal (increased heart rate) that is labeled via cognitions and then emotion (fear) is experienced. So physiological reactions must be cognitively labeled before they become emotions. Psychologist Richard Lazarus developed on this cognitive model, in 1991, with his "cognitive-meditational" model. He proposed the idea that we all have our own internal cognitive appraisals or meanings for events which for the most part remain unconscious. Following an external stimulus the amount of emotion experienced would be dependent on the individuals own cognitive appraisal. When an individual perceives something, it is the act of perception that triggers arousal and emotion.

In his 1996 book, *The Science of Emotion*, Randy Cornelius outlined the main theoretical transitions of emotion and how they have contributed to our current perspectives and understanding on the nature of emotion. The four traditions as seen by Cornelius are Darwinian, Jamesian, Cognitive, and Social Constructivist perspectives. Cornelius eloquently sums up these theoretical traditions and suggests that the Darwinian tradition posits that emotions are evolutionary and have adaptive functions. The Jamesian approach suggests that emotions arise from bodily responses. The cognitive approach looks at emotions as arising from the cognitive appraisal of a situation or event, and the Social Constructivist approach sees emotions as being social constructions that serve social purposes. Each of these perspectives offers a different way of looking at emotion, and each offers great value in understanding the nature of emotions. However, the theory that has gained most attention and prominence has been cognitive. When it comes to the practical applications in personal development and therapy, emotion is primarily viewed as a mental process that arises as a result of thinking. As we will see, the notion that emotion can be manipulated and managed simply by altering or challenging one's thought patterns is simply not an effective therapeutic method particularly when we are addressing chronic pain and fatigue symptoms.

## Origins in the Brain

In 1937 an American neuroanatomist named James Papez published a journal article outlining what he believed to be the neural pathways and brain circuitry involved in emotion. This was the first time that specific areas of the brain had been proposed as being involved in the control and production of emotion. Papez hypothesized that the hypothalamus and an area once referred to as the limbic lobe were critical. "The hypothalamus, the anterior thalamic nucleus, the cingulate gyrus, the hippocampus and their interconnections, constitute a harmonious mechanism which may elaborate the functions of central emotion as well as participate in the emotional expression."

In 1949 the "Papez Circuit" was upgraded by Yale neuroscientist Paul MacLean. MacLean was interested in where subjective experience resided in the brain and whether the circuitry of the brain had evolved over time. He suggested that a circuit consisting of the limbic lobe coupled with connections in the forebrain, including the hypothalamus, amygdala, and septum constituted what he initially called a "visceral brain," and later termed the "limbic system." The limbic system is thought to be the area of the brain that oversees emotion, memory, and arousal. The hypothalamus is a bit like the master gland of the brain, as it produces hormones, the chemical messengers that are involved in regulating a host of critical functions within the body, such as food and water levels and intake, sleep cycles, body temperature, and emotional and sexual behavior. The amygdala prepares the body for the fight-or-flight response and is involved in the formation of emotional memories that attach, or "tag," situations and circumstances.

MacLean continued his research into the evolution of the brain over time and arrived at a theory suggesting that our brains are really three brains in one—a "triune brain." In evolutionary terms, the oldest part is the reptilian brain that is responsible for basic primitive emotions such as fear and anger. The second part he described as the old "mammalian" brain or limbic system. This part builds on the primitive emotions, and is responsible for social emotions such as bonding, distress, and playfulness, as well as decoding information to give each animal its own unique experience and interpretation of life. The third part was the new "mammalian" brain, consisting of the neocortex, which interfaces brain with cognition, and exerts a top-down control over emotional responses that are driven by other systems.

MacLean's idea was that emotional experiences involve the integration of sensations from the immediate environment with information from the body. Following the William James idea, he suggested that events in the world lead to bodily changes. Information from the body informs the brain, where it is amalgamated with ongoing perceptions of current external events.

Advances in psychology and neuroscience have questioned the accuracy of the limbic model, however, it does remain a popular perspective for a basic understanding of emotion and the brain. In truth the picture is most a likely a little more complex, and different emotions correspond with different changes within the brain. But the next question is whether there is more to emotion than the activity within the brain?

## What About the Rest of the Body?

> *"Many common emotional-regulation strategies work on the*
> *assumption that all emotion follows thought, and thus, by*
> *changing one's thoughts, one should be able to gain control*
> *over one's emotions. In the last decade, however, research in*
> *neuroscience has clearly shown that intuition and emotional*

*processes operate at a much higher speed than cognitive processes. In many cases, emotions occur independently of the cognitive system and can significantly bias or color the cognitive process and its output or decision. In other words, because many emotional processes operate faster than thought processes, behaviors and decisions may be based on emotions rather than thoughtful discernment"*

—Dr. Rollin McCraty, HeartMath Institute

We often think that the brain, and specifically the thinking brain, is responsible for emotion. In fact we have seen an entire industry develop and promote books, programs, and products based on the idea that you can change the way you feel by changing the way you think, which in turn will change your life. Part of the mainstream approach to treating chronic fatigue and pain conditions is to offer cognitive behavioral therapy (CBT), with its focus on changing negative or dysfunctional thought patterns. However, it seems fairly apparent that CBT is not particularly effective in alleviating symptoms of chronic fatigue or pain, and the reasons why are beginning to emerge. Emotion is not simply the end result of thinking, it would appear that emotion involves a complex interplay of body and brain working harmoniously.

The notion of emotion being solely a byproduct of brain activity is a recent phenomenon. Ancient cultures such as the Chinese and Greeks looked to the heart as the seat of emotion, of wisdom, courage, and decision-making. Even in Western culture we place the heart as the center for passion, wisdom, and also as the center of our identity. If you stop and think about it, if you are gesturing, when talking about yourself, you would tend to point towards the center of your chest, your heart, rather than the center of your forehead.

Intuitively we know that the heart plays a significant role in our experience of life and is more than merely a muscle that pumps blood. In our everyday language there are so many phrases that make reference to the heart, or compare the heart and the head. "I should have listened to my heart not my head," or "follow your heart,"—the list of clichés goes on. But clichés come from somewhere; they have origins and meaning. Could it be that the heart actually plays a far greater role in our emotional and intuitive experience than conventional science is having us believe? The HeartMath organization in California seems to think so. Lead researcher, Dr. Rollin McCraty and his team have conducted a number of interesting experiments to demonstrate the influence of the heart on the brain. According to McCraty, the heart communicates with the brain and body in four ways: neurological communication via the nervous system, biochemical communication via the hormones, biophysical communication via pulse waves, and energetic communication via electromagnetic fields.

The team at HeartMath have also sought to measure the electric and magnetic fields produced by both the brain and the heart. They report that the heart's magnetic field is over five hundred times bigger than the brain's and that the heart's electrical field is sixty times bigger than the brain's. This effectively means that your heart fields radiate out into life, transmitting and receiving information, constantly interacting with the energy fields of other people and mass consciousness. As information travels back through the heart fields into your body, the energy is transmuted, physical changes occur and you receive feedback in the form of emotions, feelings, and intuitions. There is a strong argument to suggest that many of the subtle intuitive feelings we have arise from fluctuations within these subtle energy biofields as they detect energetic shifts in the "quantum energy soup" of life.

Not only does the heart create measurable energy fields that extend beyond the physical boundaries of your body, the heart has a mind of its own that sends meaningful messages to the brain and other areas of the body. The heart has a complex neural network, which has led scientists to refer to it as the "mini-brain." Its neural circuitry enables it to act independently of the cranial brain, to learn, remember, make decisions, and even feel and sense via the secretion of a number of hormones and neurotransmitters. There are more ascending neural pathways than descending—this essentially means that the heart sends more information to the brain than the brain sends to the heart. This gives an entirely different picture to our usual idea that intelligence takes place exclusively within the brain.

This intelligent activity within the body is not restricted to the heart. As we discussed in Chapter 2, there is a "second brain" in the gut called the enteric nervous system, and there are hundreds of millions of neurons connecting it to the cranial brain. If you have ever wondered where the term "gut feeling" comes from, or if you have ever experienced a sinking feeling in your gut, then the answer lies in the gut. It communicates with the central nervous system via the vagus nerve, which enables it to receive information, respond to emotions, and record experiences. Many gastrointestinal disorders, including colitis and irritable bowel syndrome can originate from problems within the gut's "brain"; it's the reason you experience "butterflies" in your stomach or need to use the bathroom when you are very nervous or feel "stressed."

Dr. Candace Pert pioneered the modern notion of the mind-body connection in the 1970s. While working on her PhD, she was seeking to identify opiate receptor sites, assumed to be located solely within the brain. Her research revealed that receptor sites could be found throughout the body as well as the brain. This idea proved both groundbreaking and controversial because up until this point it was assumed that intelligent activity only existed within the brain, and the body merely hosted the brain. The consensus on emotion was very "neurocentric," meaning that emotions are the result of activity within the brain. Candace Pert's work, turned this idea on its head, as she presented evidence to suggest that the body is filled with receptor sites. Once these receptors receive communication, the information cascades through the cell's interior, which triggers a number of key processes. Information flows from the brain, the heart, the gut, and the sex organs, and all over the body, resulting in something of a "conversation" of intelligent activity. The information that she spoke about came in the form of hormones, neurotransmitters, and peptides—what science refers to as a "ligand." These ligands account for almost all the data transfer throughout the body and brain, with only a small percentage resulting from synaptic activity in the brain alone.

The information transferred could be about hunger, tiredness, anger, or bliss. Dr. Pert argued that there was no difference between emotional signals and other physiological data transference—the same processes are occurring throughout the body and brain. The two components that are involved in this data transfer are the ligands—or information that flows—and the receptors found throughout the body. These are what Pert refers to as "molecules of emotion." The receptors are in a constant state of vibratory flux. A ligand that vibrates at the same frequency as a receptor site will be attracted to the receptor. When in resonance, they come together. According to Pert, "The attracting vibration is the emotion, and the actual connection—peptide to receptor—is the manifestation of feeling in the physical world. Emotions influence the molecules, which in turn is how we feel." (*Everything You Need to Know To Feel Good.* Candace B. Pert PhD 2006.)

Receptors join together in complexes forming walls and channels within cells, allowing substances to move in and out of cells creating an electrical current that moves through the body-mind. A huge amount of emotional information is channelled throughout the body and brain, and much of it remains outside conscious awareness.

Given this exciting information, it comes as no surprise that Dr. Pert defined emotion in the broadest possible way, to include common familiar emotions such as anger, fear, and joy, broad sensations of pleasure and pain, as well as the primary "drives" or motivational states such as hunger and thirst, all the way to the as yet physiologically unexplained phenomena of spiritual inspiration, awe, and bliss.

How is this important to our understanding of emotion, and how can we use this information about the physiological nature of emotion to help with symptoms of chronic pain and fatigue? We first need to understand the difference between emotions and feelings, and the implications for our health.

## What's the Difference Between Emotions and Feelings?

> "*Emotions did not evolve as conscious feeling. They evolved as behavioral and physiological specializations, as bodily responses controlled by the brain that allowed ancestral organisms to survive in hostile environments.*"
>
> —Joseph LeDoux, 1996

The idea that emotions are different from feelings may not sit well with many who often use the words emotions and feelings interchangeably, to mean largely the same thing. However, it appears that the structures involved in emotions and feelings are slightly different. Leading neurologist Antonio Damasio suggests that feelings like joy or sorrow can only emerge after the brain registers physical changes in the body. ". . . emotions are more or less the complex reactions the body has to certain stimuli. When we are afraid of something, our hearts begin to race, our mouths become dry, our skin turns pale and our muscles contract. This emotional reaction occurs automatically and unconsciously. Feelings occur after we become aware in our brain of such physical changes; only then do we experience the feeling of fear." (Scientific American April 1, 2005. *Feeling Our Emotions*.)

Emotions then could be seen as nonconscious processes occurring as a result of our ongoing interaction with the environment, while feelings could be said to be the subjective experience we have of emotions.

This is incredibly important for us in looking to understand the role of emotions in health, particularly symptoms of fatigue and pain. If we are to argue that emotions are effectively "underneath" the symptoms, it seems entirely possible that something is taking place within the body and brain whereby emotions are triggered but not felt. There's a plausible argument to suggest that with repeated unconscious suppression or blocking of emotion, a rewiring of neural pathways takes place in the brain. In effect the result of this rewiring could be that rather than triggering feelings, emotions actually trigger symptoms. This might explain our theory of the long-term stress path outlined in the previous chapter. In order to deal with the challenges of life we suppress our emotions because they are overwhelming and almost debilitating. This is not a conscious choice we make, rather it is borne out of a need to survive, to cope, to live another day. As the pattern of blocking or suppressing becomes generalized, this leads to a rewiring, whereby the structures involved in the creation of subjective feelings are not activated. With a full "stress bucket." the drip feed of additional emotion results in the subjective experience of symptoms in body and brain, via the endocrine, immune, and autonomic nervous systems.

In most instances this blocking or suppression of emotion is likely to start in childhood. As we discussed in the previous chapter, ACEs are far more common than originally thought, and lower level emotional stressors creating an ongoing negatively charged environment are almost as damaging as major traumatic events. Constant tensions between two parents creates a toxic environment as emotional energy radiates through their biofields and impacts their children. If a child is in distress or feels threatened, emotions will be triggered. If the child unconsciously senses that nothing can be done the emotions are suppressed, overridden in favor of coping. This is particularly evident when children are invited to listen to an adult and internalize what the adult is saying rather than to trust their own feelings. It is at this stage that the development of a lack of trust of one's own feelings takes place.

As a father of two daughters when my children were very young I was extremely aware of the language I used and the extent to which I encouraged them to validate their own feeling experience. I was also struck by how easy it is for parents to tell their children how they should feel or even how they do feel, especially when the parent is seeking to minimize their own internal discomfort. How often have you heard a parent tell a young child to stop crying, or tell them they do like something when the child is trying to state otherwise. These repeated patterns can seem harmless but over time lead to a distrust of and detachment from one's own feelings. Of course in instances where abuse has taken place of one form or another the detachment from feeling can happen almost immediately.

Blocking emotion is reasonably easy for most of us because it is our cognitive or thinking brain that controls our conscious attention. When emotion is overwhelming or believed to be a hindrance, attention and energy can reside solely in the thinking brain, effectively cutting off feedback from the emotional brain and body. In his highly readable book, *Healing Without Freud or Prozac*, psychiatrist, Dr. David Servan-Schreiber, describes an experiment aimed at identifying and mapping areas of the brain involved in emotional experiences. The experiment involved showing disturbing videos to subjects while monitoring their brain's activity using an MRI scanner (magnetic resonance imaging) as well as measuring heart rate and blood pressure. During an experimental session with one female participant, Servan-Schreiber could see that her blood pressure and her heart rate were worryingly elevated. Concerned that she was experiencing a great deal of stress, he went into the lab and asked if she was okay, and if she wanted him to turn off the video and end the session. She looked at him with an element of surprise on her face and said she was completely fine, couldn't feel anything and was quite happy to continue viewing. In his book, Servan-Schreiber suggests that the lady was detached from her emotional feelings and therefore was not particularly emotionally intelligent. He goes on to say that as a researcher at the university she was seen by colleagues as cold and aloof. I would go somewhat further and suggest that this is a great example of the difference between emotion and feeling and how it is entirely possible to block and suppress our emotion when we get stuck in our thinking brain. The result is that our "head" or cognitive brain can think one thing while our intelligent body, which includes the emotional brain, can have an entirely different opinion. This lady in the experiment reported feeling fine even though her body was showing significant signs of stress. The risk for her is that without awareness of her intelligent body and the feeling feedback it offers, she lacks the ability to detect when her body is in a long-term state of stress. This, as we now know can ultimately lead to irregularities within body systems and the appearance of symptoms and disease. Reconnecting the thinking brain and the intelligent body is a vital element in recovering from a chronic fatigue or pain condition as well as maintaining optimum health and performance. As long as a fracture remains between these two parts of us the flow of communication remains disrupted and we are unable to fully attune to and align with our true self.

## Where Does Emotion Come From and Can It Be Changed?

We can now see that emotion is a complex physiological process that involves all of the body and all of the brain and is not different from other basic physiological drives such as hunger and tiredness. Paying attention to feeling feedback like the pain that arises when there is a stone in our shoe, the rumbling feeling that accompanies hunger, and the variety of sensations that let us know our body is tired, probably seem relatively straightforward and will certainly become easier the more you pay attention. When the stone is in our shoe we take it out, when the body sends those hunger signals the only decision we have to make is what to eat. When the body sends healthy tired signals we just have to work out when we can have a nap or get to bed. (I am making a distinction here between healthy tired and a symptom of fatigue, which is usually an uncomfortable groggy feeling. As we will see later, symptoms of fatigue are not a sign to rest, they are a sign that there is an emotional buildup of frustrated boredom.) However, when it comes to emotion the picture gets a little more complex. We tend to judge and resist our emotion or try to resolve it by analyzing it and ourselves. There isn't necessarily one action, one set of words, one direction or solution. But before we get into how we figure all that out, we need to understand where our emotion comes from so we can understand exactly what we need to do with it. There have been emotional researchers who have sought to classify emotions in certain ways, and for many years in my practice I would talk about primary and secondary emotions, then core and mind emotions, but ultimately what we need is not additional layers of complexity, rather we need something very straightforward that we can understand and work with.

We have learned that emotion is a nonconscious process and somewhat different from feelings, which we are aware of. Understanding emotion from a scientific and academic perspective is certainly interesting and offers us some valuable insights. However, what is vitally important for you reading this book is to have a practical understanding of emotion so that you can acknowledge it, feel it, process, and regulate it in order to prevent it from building up in your stress bucket.

Your emotions arise as a result of your interaction with your environment. That means whatever you do, whatever you say, how you act in this moment, how you approach whatever you are doing, all contributes to your current emotional experience. The meaning of your emotion is to guide you back to your true self. This is why when we are aligned with our true self our emotional our experience seems more stable than when we are not. Your emotion is about you, it is feedback to you about what you are doing and whether your actions are aligned with your true self. The further you are from your true self the greater the negative emotional experience you will experience. Your emotional experience is never really about other people, it is about you, even though we often want to blame others for how we feel. As you align your actions with your true self your intelligent body reduces the amount of negative emotion that you experience. When we look at emotion from this perspective it is extremely empowering. It means that we can take responsibility for what we do and what we say.

Let's look at a simple example of this: If your boss suggests that a piece of work you have done is not good enough, you might experience some negative emotion in the form of hurt and anger. Your actions immediately following this will impact significantly what happens to that hurt and anger. If you run and hide in the stationery closet you might find there is an amplification of your hurt and anger, especially if your mind becomes involved and more emotions are triggered. If you go back and review your work, identify how it could be improved, and set about making the changes you feel are the right ones for you, your hurt and anger could be transformed into positive, higher vibrational emotions— this is constructive action.

So our emotional experience literally unfolds in front of us, as we interact with everything and everyone around us. Changes in our emotional experience usually arise when we change the nature of our interaction with the environment. If you're wondering exactly what I mean by "environment," it is simply everything that you come into contact with: people, places, and things that you do. We are always in contact or interacting with something, even if we are lying down in a dark room. If we are alive, we are engaged in an activity within an environment.

We can often fall into the trap of thinking we are passive observers of life, that everything outside of us triggers our emotions and there's nothing we can do about it. This is not the case. We are in fact active players in our own game of life. Everything we do and say has an energetic impact and influence. So, we are far from being the emotional victims of circumstance; we play an enormous role in our own ongoing emotional experience. A useful way to consider emotions is that their role is to guide us in certain directions. They are a call to action, in much the same way as lights on a car dashboard invite us to act. The key is that we need to take action in the present (don't worry if this doesn't quite make sense yet—

there is much more about how to do this as we move through the rest of the book).

Emotion is an energy that needs to flow. The source of that energy can be *internal*; this could be a transduction of energy—a change of energy from one form to another arising inside of us. Or it can be our body responding to *external* energies within our environment. Through our heart field or biofield, we transmit and receive energy; we exert an influence and are influenced by the energies within our environment.

Let's begin by looking at these two sources in more detail, internal and external. First, the internal:

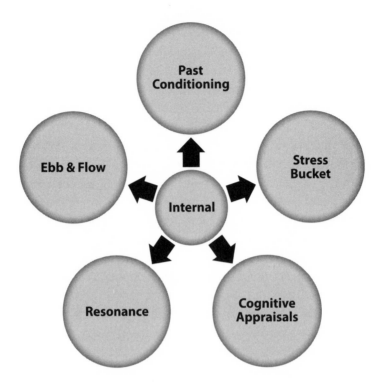

1. PAST CONDITIONING. We have seen from psychology and neuroscience that a huge amount of our emotion comes from learned experience. Situations are "tagged" with emotional markers and these emotions are triggered when we encounter similar situations or experiences. These emotions and resulting feelings arise internally, meaning that they are not directly "caused" by external situations; rather it is our intelligent body's response to external events based on past experience and our current "resonance" in this moment (we'll come back to resonance, below). The notion of past experience and conditioning is familiar to most people; so, if you have a negative experience in a certain situation that situation is emotionally "tagged" by your nervous system. Next time you encounter the same or similar circumstances you will experience some of the same emotions as a reminder that the previous experience was unpleasant. If your second exposure to the same situation is positive then the negative emotion subsides and is overlaid with positive emotion. When you come into contact with that situation for the

third time your initial feeling experience is far less negative. Consistent positive experience will in effect override the initial emotional tags. There is an argument to suggest that the markers of these initial experiences never actually go away, they are just overlaid with new emotional markers, almost like laying blankets on top of one another.

2. THE STRESS BUCKET. In the last chapter, we talked about how emotion can build up in our stress bucket. This can happen over a prolonged period of time, or over a very short period of time. The emotion that is "sitting" in our stress bucket affects our perceptions of existing events. Let's use an example: Bob has a frustrating day at the office, sales have fallen through and several customers have complained that their orders have not arrived in time. Bob feels pretty helpless because he's taking the brunt of customer frustrations even though he was not at fault. He leaves the office and internalizes his feelings, shoving them deep down inside. His head begins to go into overdrive and his negative emotions increase. On the drive home, somehow he manages to find himself almost crashing, which just adds insult to injury. When Bob arrives home, he switches off the car, walks up the driveway and opens the front door. His dog, Bonzo, comes bounding over and jumps up to greet Bob. "Get down Bonzo, you bad dog." shouts Bob, his frustrations finally spilling over.

The notion of spilling over is interesting, especially as what we are witnessing here is Bob's stress bucket filling up reasonably quickly. The emotions he had experienced and probably suppressed earlier in the day affect the emotional feelings he experiences at the end of the day—it's as if they are all sloshing around together in his stress bucket. On a different day Bob would have responded in an entirely different way to Bonzo, giving him a big hug rather than a scolding. Again, this idea of emotion building up until finally we explode like a volcanic eruption is probably familiar to you. One of the biggest problems with this boom-and-silence approach to processing emotion is that when the volcano of emotion erupts most people feel guilt and think they are too emotional or have an anger problem. In truth, what is actually happening is that short-term emotional suppression is leading to a full stress bucket. Constructive action on emotional feelings as they arise can prevent this buildup.

3. COGNITIVE APPRAISALS. Much of our emotional experience comes from the meaning we imprint upon the world. Academics call these the "unconscious appraisals" we make of situations and events. External events do not possess any inherent meaning in and of themselves; it is only the meaning we imprint upon them. If you were to stop for a moment and think about a sport that you like, maybe you love football or tennis. When you watch a game on television there's a strong chance that you will be rooting for one team or player in the game. In fact, you're probably thinking about this right now as you're reading. As you think about it, you may even get a hint of the emotion you felt during the last game you watched. As I am sure you can appreciate, there is no inherent meaning in the game, the meaning is imprinted by you. The only way you can have this emotional experience when watching a game is if at some level you have unconsciously "decided" that the outcome of the match matters—this meaning comes from inside you. You would find it very hard to change the emotion you experience by thinking about it, in much the same way as you didn't consciously decide that the match was going to mean something to you and therefore you experienced emotion. Our emotion is not controlled by our conscious thought. With that in mind, you may be wondering whether it is possible to manipulate or change emotional experiences. The simple answer is that it is, to a degree. As we will go on to see later in the book, our focus, attention, and behavior play an enormous role in the creation and experience of emotion. So it is very often the case that we are having a huge impact on our emotional experience without even realizing it.

Going back to our sporting event, if you are wondering why there is so much emotion involved in simply being a spectator, then the answer is that arguably, in the absence of meaning life would be bland and boring. There would be nothing to color our experience—in fact there would be no experience, simply data. There would be nothing to motivate us, nothing to drive us or give us reasons for engaging with the world around us. So we should welcome our emotion exactly because it is what turns a situation or event into an actual experience.

Are there any downsides to this? Well, emotional experience is wonderful, however, when this experience becomes overly negative and excessive, we step into the realm of drama. Drama arises from imprinting a significant amount of emotion onto an event, often purely for the experience of having emotion. Is there a problem with this? Arguably no. At our core we desire experience, and some experience is better than no experience. This is not dissimilar from a child acting-up or being naughty and the parent suggesting that this is for the purposes of gaining or seeking attention. The idea being that having negative attention is better than not having any attention at all. Emotion can work in a very similar fashion as we grow up into adulthood. Even though it is generally assumed that we will do what we can to avoid uncomfortable emotion and do what we can to seek pleasant emotion, in the absence of any experience we can often gravitate towards drama, because this provides an experience, even though it may not be the most pleasant or seemingly beneficial one. Here's a great example, a while back I was reading the newspaper and a headline caught my eye, it read, *Shocking but true: students prefer jolt of pain to being made to sit and think*. The researchers had subjects sit in a room alone and do nothing. That meant no reading, no phones, and no sleeping, just being alone with their thoughts for a period of 6 to 15 minutes. The general view following this was that the experience was tedious and miserable, so the researchers added an extra dimension to the experiment. They gave the research subjects the option of administering a small electric shock to themselves during the time when they were sitting doing nothing. Much to the surprise of the research team, 12 out of 18 men and 6 out of 24 women gave themselves as many as four electric shocks. What's even more amazing is that these very same people had said before the start of the experiment that they would pay to avoid being given an electric shock after having a demonstration.

While this may seem somewhat amusing to think that people would opt to give themselves an uncomfortable electric shock rather than just sit in silence, it emphasizes the point that some experience is preferable to no experience. Drama is much the same and while there is no problem in and of itself in us creating drama in order to gain an emotional experience, what is important is that we take responsibility for it. Problems can ensue when we allow ourselves to be disempowered, assume drama simply happens to us, yet we become addicted to the emotional fix it gives us because there is no other significant emotional experience in our lives.

Thinking or assuming that drama is happening to us and that our emotion lies beyond our control is misguided. We need to recognize that our emotion is coming from inside us, created by us, not the event itself, because emotion is what gives life flavor, texture, color, and meaning. When we do this we can remove blame and judgment from events or people. The students in the experiment were in complete control of their experience, so there was no option to blame anyone else. When drama comes knocking, the tendency is to blame everyone and everything else.

4. RESONANCE. While the previous three points seem fairly obvious and are probably not new, resonance is something that you may not be familiar with. When we are in "resonance" with our true self, our vibration is higher, we feel good, our head is uncluttered, and life seems to flow. As we become misaligned with our true self our vibration drops and we fall out of resonance with our true self (I'll go into greater detail in the next chapter). When we are out of resonance with our true self we tend to experience, among other things, greater emotional fluctuations. I'm sure you've had the experience of noticing that one day you experience a huge amount of emotion about something small, like your colleague leaving the milk out of the fridge in the office kitchen, then a few days later experience far less emotion in relation to a similar incident. Even though we think that our emotion is caused by these external events, the amount of emotion we feel is massively impacted by the extent to which we are aligned with our true self.

While we do play a significant role in influencing the extent to which we are aligned and in resonance, there is also a natural ebb and flow to energy and life. Sometimes this ebb and flow can seem cyclic, other times is can appear random. Our moods change and often move in cycles. Sometimes we feel upbeat and on top of the world for seemingly no reason, while other times we may feel in a lower mood and off kilter. It maybe that there is no immediately apparent reason for this. These shifts in how we feel impact our emotional responses to the world around us. Recognizing this can help us to redirect our focus from external events to internal feelings. This is not to say we are not impacted by external events, because we most certainly are. However, when we give responsibility for how we feel exclusively to external events and circumstances we disempower ourselves and move further away from true self alignment.

Have you ever had that experience where a family member does something, and your intelligent body sends you some emotion that we could call anger? As you blame them and attribute your feelings to their actions you seem to experience even more anger, even more irritation. Then a few days later the same thing happens again but this time you don't really register that there has been a difference in how you feel?

We can't extricate ourselves from our environment. Energetically, we are intertwined with it and each other, so we are always going to be impacted by the energy of life and others, as we'll see in more detail below. However, knowing that our emotional experience is not directly caused by events and people can be extremely useful and empowering, and it will make a significant impact on your behavior. When you think something has "made" you angry, you become a "victim" and you act like a "victim." Your body produces more anger in response, not because you are a victim, but ironically because at your core your true self knows that you are not a victim, and your body is using stronger and stronger feelings to get your attention and have you align with your true self, with home base. Emotional feelings are guiding you back to your true self. More negative emotion often means we are straying further from our true self, almost as we are walking a path that is taking us further and further away from that home base. The emotions are trying to pull us back on track and have us act from our true self space. When we take responsibility for our feelings it doesn't mean that we can control what we feel in this now moment because we can't; however, we can affect our ongoing emotional experience by directing our words and actions and minimizing our disruptive thinking patterns.

We are responsible for whether our emotion flows or becomes blocked and suppressed. Our tendency to blame external events, suggesting that our emotion is "caused" by them, leads us down a path where we give up our ability to effectively process our emotion and modify our behavior.

5. YOUR INNATE "WIRING." This forms the foundation for your feeling experience. It is different from the academic notion of personality, which is somewhat more complex and arguably fluid. For the purposes of simplicity and ease when working with emotional feelings, we are going to entertain the notion that your innate wiring accounts for those feeling experiences that tend not to change significantly over time. Since we cannot control our emotional feelings as they

arise our aim is to acknowledge, allow, act on, and process them, without resistance and without judgment. As you evolve and grow your feeling feedback will change to reflect the developing you. As your vibration shifts your emotional experience will change. The perspective we want to adopt is to be open to the idea that what we feel in this moment is a representation of who we are in this moment. We want to avoid falling into the trap of clutching to an idea or conception of who we are and then try to fit our emotional experience to that idea of who we are.

You might be wondering why we have not covered thinking and the role it plays in our emotional experience. There are two reasons for this; first, we are going to be covering thinking in Chapter 6, The Expanded Self; second, while thinking plays a role in our emotional experience, it is important to emphasize that much of our thinking is influenced by our emotion, so our focus is on directing attention to emotion rather than focusing on challenging thinking patterns.

Now we've covered the internal factors, let's have a little look at the external triggers.

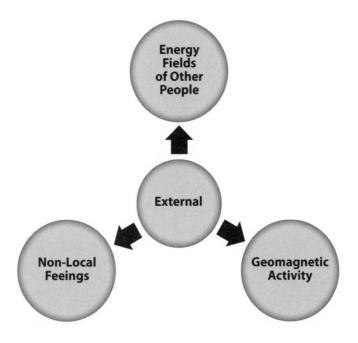

Human beings are both receivers and transmitters of energy. We possess an energetic sensitivity that enables us to detect energetic changes around us. The word "energy" may seem a little "out there" and arguably it is. Hard scientists tend to get a little irritated and think that the meaning of energy is misappropriated or misinterpreted. However, I would argue that the notion of subtle energies is prevalent in Eastern traditions and it is only in the West that we hold onto the notion that if we can't measure it doesn't exist. We have already uncovered that the heart creates and regulates electric and magnetic fields that can be measured and form something of a biofield around the body. These energies may well be accompanied by other subtle energies that we have yet to detect but that still impact our experience of life.

Let's look in a little more detail at those external energies that impact our emotional experience.

1. THE ENERGY FIELDS OF OTHER PEOPLE. Have you ever had the experience of walking into a party or social event and immediately feeling or sensing the atmosphere? Or maybe, you could feel it as you were approaching? As individuals we radiate energy through our biofield, and we detect other people's energy in much the same way. The more empathic you are the more sensitive you are to the energy and vibration emitted by other people. One of the difficulties for the empath is knowing when the feelings they are experiencing are theirs, or the result of detecting someone else's "emissions," so to speak. There is absolutely nothing wrong with detecting other people's energy, in fact I would suggest that sensitivity is a strength, not a weakness as many people think. Sensitivity describes the ability to detect, and I would encourage you to embrace your sensitivity. I can certainly speak from experience; growing up, I believed my sensitivity was something to bury deep down. Being a sensitive male was not something to talk about. But in suppressing this truth about myself, I was denying myself, abandoning the truth of who I was. Whether you are male or female, open up and find the strengths in your sensitivity; know that it gives you a connection to others and an ability to form deep connections.

Some people's sensitivity extends to being able to detect recent historical emotional energy. I remember a client telling me that she could feel the emotional energy in places after those who had radiated that energy had left. She once told me about going to a restaurant and feeling a sense of agitation or discomfort as she was shown to her table. This contrasted the pleasant body feelings she had experienced only moments earlier. When she asked the waiter about the previous patrons, he told her that a couple had been at the table and had a blazing argument, with both visibly angry. One had stormed out, closely followed by the other. The energy they both radiated remained almost like an imprint in the quantum soup, waiting to be detected.

Go back to our sporting example earlier when you were to imagine being in the stadium watching a match. Even with little or no interest in the outcome, you would feel the energy of the crowd and this would undoubtedly impact your emotional experience. If you had imprinted meaning onto the outcome of the match, then you would have the dual impact of your own meaning-based emotion, plus the energy of the crowd.

2. GEOMAGNETIC SENSITIVITY is the ability to detect changes coming from within the earth and environment before they happen. An example of this being where people can feel or sense when an earthquake is about to occur. Energetically, this remains largely unexplained, however, it is scientifically demonstrable.

Many people will be affected by changes in atmospheric pressure, or sudden weather changes, as well as lunar cycles. An article called "The Dark Side Of The Moon," published in the *Medical Journal of Australia* in 2009, described how the number of women admitted to hospital for overdose dropped significantly around the time of a full moon, while men were more likely to overdose at that time. The conclusion of the research was: "Violent and acute behavioral disturbance manifested more commonly during the full moon." Michel Gauquelin, the French psychologist, identified a significant link between the position of the moon and career choice. He posited that writers and politicians tended to be born when the moon was at the highest point in the sky, or when it was rising. He then extended his research and found that the positions of Saturn and Mars were influential as well. Correlation doesn't imply causation, however these are certainly interesting findings.

The value in recognizing the impact of external energies is that it enables us to make sense of our feeling experience, so we can identify the triggers of feeling states and then begin to take appropriate action where needed. As we have an extreme tendency to analyze and resist our feeling experience, when we recognize the origins of that experience we can begin to allow it to flow through us without comment, attached meaning, or resistance.

3. NONLOCAL FEELINGS. These fall more into the category of intuitions (see below), and are where a feeling is present that connects to a person or event in a different location. An example being where a mother senses something about a child many miles away. This sort of experience is an example of what quantum theorists describe as quantum entanglement, or "action at a distance." Arguably it is not distinctly different from telepathy or clairvoyance, however it is a very real and measurable phenomenon. These feelings, like intuitions, can present themselves as inner "knowings" or as actual body sensations. Either way, they are not something we can, or would want to change. They are extremely valuable feedback, and reinforce the energetic nature of life.

As we can see certain aspects of our emotional experience can and will change, while others will not. What is important to remember is that our emotional experience is fluid—an energy in motion that needs to flow—and given the opportunity it will resolve itself. It's also worth bearing in mind that because our emotional experience is fluid it can be influenced by many factors and the way we feel about things can depend on the context, as well as the other emotions present in our body and mind at the time.

## High and Low Vibrational Emotions

A simple Google search requesting a list of emotions shows that there are well over a hundred English words to describe different emotions. The same search reveals that there are a variety of ways of categorizing emotions, as well including simple emotions, complex emotions, and pure emotions. However, as we are defining emotion as a vibrational energy in motion, we are going to use a very basic categorization of low vibrational emotions and high vibrational emotions. Low (or negative) vibrational emotions tend to be incoherent or distorted in their energy patterns. They can lead to a constricting of the braiding of your DNA, and impact the functioning of the cells of the body and brain. This makes them disruptive to body systems which means that when they are in excess or blocked they can cause a triggering of body symptoms. High (or positive) vibrational emotions are coherent in their energy patterns. They facilitate effective functioning within body systems and thus improve health and well-being—this effectively means that when positive emotions are present within body and brain it is extremely unlikely that body symptoms will increase. The list below is not exhaustive, but gives an indication of the different emotions.

| HIGH VIBRATIONAL (POSITIVE) EMOTIONS | LOW VIBRATIONAL (NEGATIVE) EMOTIONS |
|---|---|
| Love and Compassion | Anger |
| Joy | Fear (including worry and concern) |
| Happiness | Boredom* (lack of joy) |
| Excitement | Frustration and Agitation |
| Bliss | Sadness/Grief |
| Satisfaction | Disgust |

*Boredom refers to a lack of fulfillment or joy in the present moment. It is possible to be very busy and still very bored. Don't fall into the trap of thinking that just because you are occupied you are not bored.

For our purposes, a simple categorization of high and low vibration, or positive and negative, will suffice. Our emotional feeling experience is often an amalgamation of different emotions, so attempting to unpick exactly what we feel is not particularly productive, and tends to result in excessive analysis. Our goal is not to transcend our negative emotions. Our aim is to fully feel our emotions and allow them to guide us back to our true self. Our emotions present our truth in this now moment, despite the tendency to want to delve into past events. We cannot change our emotional experience now by analyzing the past. Emotions are a tap on the shoulder inviting us to align our words and actions with our true self in this now moment. I don't think this is necessarily an easy concept to embrace, so we will return to it frequently throughout the book and look at it from different angles, to help you embed it as a principle.

## Intuition and Inner Knowing

*If emotion is our intelligent body's way of inviting us to align with our true self, intuition and inner knowing could be said to be direct communication from that true self.*

Intuition is the inner guidance we experience but can't seem to explain—when we feel a push or a pull towards or away from certain things. Sometimes we just seem to know things and can't explain why or how. It is different from emotion but equally if not more important as a tool to help us navigate through life. Intuition is communication from our true self, and it can present through physical feelings, thoughts, or ideas that just seem to pop into your head, a flow of energy that is moving through you, or simply a deep inner knowing. This level of feeling is subtle and needs to be developed and nurtured through trust. Because of its subtle nature, intuition can be drowned out by the cacophony of mental chatter that develops the more time we spend in our head. However, the more you trust and act on intuitive nudges and knowings, the stronger they become. Internal conflict often arises when your intuition is nudging you in one direction and your thinking is trying to pull you in another direction. I am inviting you to believe that the intuition is guidance from your true self, whereas thinking, despite being a valid part of your experience, does not represent your true self. Your thinking is more like a machine that collects and collates information from external sources and then spews it into your consciousness. In many instances this is helpful, but when there is a conflict between this thinking and your intuition I would encourage you to trust and act on your intuition first.

The scientific perspective suggests that intuition is the ability to assimilate and process information in ways that exceed the speed and capacity of normal cognitive processing. This information processing is taking place all the time outside of conscious awareness and is perceived by the body's psychophysiological systems. Because intuition can present itself as body feelings there is something of an overlap between emotion and intuition. However, they are different. Sometimes it is possible for emotions to present themselves, while at the same time there are intuitions or inner knowings underneath. For example, if you were faced with a situation whereby you had an option to leave your job and take different job or line of work. You feel scared because there are so many unknowns and you think the feeling of scared is encouraging you to run away from this option as fast as possible. But underneath that scared there is an intuition that is pulling you towards the new job. You can't explain it, but somehow you know that the intuition is right. The emotion is useful and valuable and it is not in opposition to your intuition. This is why it can so valuable to understand that emotion is guiding you back to your true self and intuition is direct communication from your true self. The emotion in this example is there to protect you, to ensure that you are not careless or cavalier.

Another important distinction for us to make is between instinct and intuition. Often the words instinct and intuition are used interchangeably, but there is a subtle difference. Instinct is a fairly fixed pattern of behavior that you might have as a human being in response to a certain stimulus or situation. Intuition is communication from your true self. In the main, paying attention to instinct is usually of value; however, there are times when just blindly following instinct is not always the best option. A good example of this is where feelings are concerned. Our natural instinct when experiencing negative feelings is to get away from them as quickly as possible. This could be through resistance and burying or could be though a behavior such as lashing out or aggression. However, moving to a higher level of consciousness and allowing ourselves to experience our feelings helps us develop and evolve. Instinct can feel like a reaction or an impulse, while intuition is a deeper feeling like an energy moving through you. As you begin to pay attention to what takes place in your body you'll find that you can begin to distinguish between all these forms of feedback.

CHAPTER 4

# Energy-flow: Key Principles

THERE IS AN ARGUMENT TO SUGGEST THAT FOR MANY things in life it is not necessary for us to understand how something works in order to derive benefit from it. Knowing and understanding exactly how your TV works certainly won't add anything to your viewing experience. The same could be said for some healthcare treatments and procedures where you don't play an active role in the process of recovery. For example, if you needed shoulder surgery following an accident, you don't need to know exactly how the orthopedic surgeon will do what he does in the operating theater.

However, this work is different. Even though there are various exercises that pepper this book, Energy-flow Coaching™ is not a series of techniques that you put into practice in a stepwise manner. It is more like a body of knowledge that you need to understand and integrate. There are some exercises that fall out of that knowledge, but they are just designed to nudge you along the path to greater understanding and alignment with your true self. This book is offering you a perspective on how you work, how you function as a human being. When you embrace that understanding it enables you to take charge of yourself, your health, and your own destiny.

As we move through this guidebook we are going to return and make reference to a number of ideas and concepts that will help you implement the principles and practices. If at any stage of the book you are confused then you can return to this chapter and remind yourself of the key foundational principles. These principles form the basis of every other aspect of the book.

Many of the subsections of the Energy-flow Coaching™ model may at first glance seem familiar to those with knowledge of personal

development and therapy, such as boundary setting, effective communication, and meeting needs. However, there are unique elements
to both the definition and approach to dealing with these areas, so
adopting a "beginner's mind" will be useful. In working with clients
over the last 15 years I have had many express to me that they've
"heard it all before," through books and other therapeutic modalities,
only to recant, as the differences in this work become a little more
apparent. Adopting a beginner's mind is incredibly difficult because
as human beings we are designed to learn quickly and move forward
with that learning. In saying that, it is possible to sit with this material
and allow yourself to feel into it, holding an intention that you are
open to new understandings and new learnings despite being familiar with some of the words and phrases used.

I've already talked about your true self in sections of this book, so
we'll begin our Key Principles by delving into what that is and what
it isn't.

## Your True Self

At your core there is a vibrational frequency or inner wisdom that is
your true self. This frequency extends beyond the physical boundaries of your body and radiates into the energetic quantum soup of life.
This true self is the real you, and it needs to flow freely and experience itself in order for you to enjoy health and vitality. This true self
is not fixed. It is fluid; it cannot be caged or defined, it needs to be
emancipated and experienced. You receive energy from the environment all around, and you transmit light, energy, and vibration, which
impacts upon everything you come into contact with. So your very
existence exerts an energetic and vibrational influence, which has an
impact on your experience of life and your conception of reality.

The idea of a true self may seem a little bizarre despite it being
such a commonly used phrase in the worlds of health, personal development, and spirituality. It suggests that there is part of you that is
the real you, which means there must be other parts that are not the
real you—but how does that work? One thing is for sure, thinking
and analyzing are not going to help on the road to experiencing your
true self. I have had many clients over the years say to me, "But what
if I don't like the real me," or, "How do I find my authentic self." If
you notice yourself asking these questions it is an indicator that you

are in your "head" and that is not where you'll find the answer. If you allow your thinking brain to go searching for who you are, you could find yourself tumbling down a rabbit hole of confusion and endless introspection. In fact, I'd go so far as to say that you don't need to know intellectually, and as soon as you try to define yourself from that intellectual space you are already limiting who you might be; you are putting yourself in a box.

I'd like you to imagine yourself as having a frequency, almost like your own radio station that you can tune into. This frequency has a rhythm and vibration. You know when you are tuned-in because you feel good, life seems to flow and your outlook is more positive. This is when you are in your Energy-flow; you are aligned with your true self and your vibration is high. You may have come across the word "flow" or term "flow-state" to refer to when you are in peak performance, at the top of your game. The term "flow" is used most frequently to describe the experience someone might have during a high-risk sport, or some other activity where there is a meshing of mind and body, cognitive and physiological, to maximize performance. Your Energy-flow is different. Energy-flow describes a state of being where you are aligned with your core frequency, you are tuned into the emotions and intuitions that your intelligent body sends and your words and actions flow from your true self. It does not describe your performance externally in the world as such; it describes an internal experience that arises from alignment with your true self.

Your true self is not something you can grasp cognitively or mentally because it is expansive and free flowing and has the capacity to change. Your mind will desperately want to jump in and try and figure out who you are and keep you locked in a very tight definition of yourself. It will look back at who you have been in the past and want to project that out into the future. This egoic-mind wants to protect you and keep you safe; however, in doing so it tends to view everything from a perspective of fear or scarcity, clutching to the familiar and resisting difference or change. The egoic-mind serves a valuable purpose in some regard in that we do maintain a degree of consistency in our identity rather than going insane by being radically different from moment to moment. However, this same egoic-mind can be hugely restricting by deciding who we are without factoring in our capacity to change and flow. Who we are is constantly shifting and changing, we are an energy in flow, we are not something frozen in time, despite the apparent safety in this option. When we allow our egoic-mind to run the show we begin to deviate from our true self because we tend to put ourselves in a box; we think we know who we are while in truth we are probably out of touch. As we will go on and see, our sense of identity is a very powerful motivator or controller of our behavior, even if that sense of identify is different from our true self. This is where it becomes important to nurture and develop self-awareness, releasing the hold of the egoic-mind, letting go of the idea that you absolutely know who you are, and beginning to open up to the possibility that there is more to you than you currently know.

*Could you entertain the idea of being curious about who you might be; letting go of having to know who you are?*

I often encourage my clients to, "Be curious about who you might be," because it is only when we let go of trying to figure ourselves out, or trying to hold on to a rigid sense of identity that we really begin to experience who we are and who we can be. This is when we are aligned with our true self and experience our Energy-flow. We have the capacity to be many different versions or aspects having experiences at different times. You could a joker, a storyteller, a healer, a footballer, a ballerina, a wallflower, a leader, a follower. Opening up to the possibility that there are many aspects of you is opening up to feeling and letting the true self flow.

So our true self is not some absolute that we can define, it is an experience we have in a moment in time. There are aspects to it and those aspects can manifest themselves as we tune-in to our core frequency, feel, and set ourselves free. The only way you can be curious about who you might be is to be aware, to observe, not with a laser like cognitive focus that will draw you into thinking, but rather an expansive, playful awareness. Your true self will communicate via your intelligent body with intuitive feelings, knowings, gentle nudges that pull you in a particular direction. Pay attention to these subtle feelings and nudges and let your actions be guided by them.

*Emotional feelings are inviting you to align with your true self and intuition is direct communication from your true self.*

You will have experienced this communication from your true self; it's part of who you are. Even if you feel disconnected or out of touch, the communication is there under the surface. It's easy to get caught up in your head, thinking and analyzing, all the while your true self is doing its best to guide you with its subtle feedback and wisdom. When you start attuning more frequently to your true self you will notice that the decisions you make are better for you—in fact you'll find it easier to make decisions when in alignment because you will be clearer about what you want. Your mind will be less cluttered and life will generally seem better. You are likely to experience fewer symptoms and the emotions you experience will flow through you more readily.

The good news is that your natural tendency is to be in alignment with your true self, almost as if this is your default setting. There will be times when you feel good and times when you don't feel so good, the key is to recognize where you are on the spectrum. The more aligned we are with our true self the more we experience a state of high vibrational consciousness. The more misaligned we are the more we experience a state of low consciousness. The table below represents the two extremes of the spectrum. As we go through each day our tendency will be to move up and down the spectrum. As you implement the principles and practices in this book you will naturally find yourself moving back into alignment with your true self and therefore high vibrational consciousness; not through force or focus, rather through feeling and allowing.

### The Impact of Emotion

When aligned with your true self you flow more easily, but this does not mean that you are going to be happy all the time. Happiness is an emotion, just like sadness, joy, or anger. As we talked about in the previous chapter, emotions are part of the human experience; they are neither good nor bad. We cannot escape them or transcend them—it is what we do with them, how we respond that is important. Our emotional experience will shift and change over time, but we do not consciously control it as such. When we are in an Energy-flow and aligned with true self, we can experience the full range of emotions in a "healthy" way, meaning they don't get stuck, blocked, or out of balance. We can pay attention to our emotional feedback and recognize that its job is to guide us, not to block us. Emotion shines the light that illuminates the path back to our true self. As we experience a high consciousness state our thoughts, words, and actions will be more compassionate and considered. Conversely, low consciousness brings with it a tendency to react in an impulsive or hostile manner.

When our intelligent body "sends" negative emotion we tend to wobble like a Weeble. It can feel as if we have moved out of alignment with our true self because we feel off-kilter, we feel uncomfortable. But feeling low vibrational emotions is part of the experience of being human and it doesn't mean that we are disconnected from our true self. When we resist the discomforts that can accompany

| High Consciousness — Aligned With True Self | Low Consciousness — Misaligned With True Self |
| --- | --- |
| Symptom free | Symptomatic |
| Feel connected and at peace | Feel disconnected and off-kilter |
| Clear mind | Cluttered mind |
| Higher level performance/you are on top of your game | Performance drops as mind gets busier |
| Life seems to flow | Life is an uphill struggle |
| Feel good about yourself & life | Don't feel good about yourself |
| Compassionate outlook | Negative or hostile outlook |
| Experience emotional stability | Experience emotional instability |
| Good things just seem to happen | Bad things seem to happen |
| Seeking solutions | Stuck in problems |
| High level of trust of intuition | Ignore intuition, tendency to over think everything |
| Decision making is easy and effective | Decision making is difficult and often turns out badly |

low vibrational emotions, our thinking brain springs into action as it tries to find meaning, analyze, resolve, or solve our low vibrational emotion. This amplifies our wobbling and our immediate experience becomes more uncomfortable and more thinking and negative emotion ensues. This can lead to a spiraling down the vibrational spectrum. To avoid this, follow these steps:

- Acknowledge the emotion and allow it.
- Stay with the physical sensations of the emotion and avoid getting pulled into the thinking brain.
- Recognize that your emotions are never a problem and are just inviting you to act authentically in that moment.
- Take constructive and considered action if it is appropriate or just feel your feelings if that is all that needs to be done.
- If you feel very affected by the low vibrational emotion and can sense you have slipped down the spectrum, pause and remember that you can allow the feeling to flow through you and when you move back to higher consciousness you will be better placed to make decisions or take action based on what you want or what is right for you.

When you follow these steps the emotional energy will flow through you. This is processing and regulating your emotion in action. When we do this we wobble for a short period then return back to our default setting. Even though it can feel as if we are slipping way down the vibrational spectrum we are simply wobbling a little. Being aligned and in a high vibrational space does not mean that we don't experience low vibrational emotion. It does not mean that we are in a perennial state of bliss. Our very nature as human beings means that we will experience the full range of moods and emotions, and we can remain in high vibrational consciousness while experiencing all emotions. However, if those low vibrational emotions and feelings of discomfort move from being acute to chronic, or from mild to severe, you know you are slipping down into low consciousness.

## Low Consciousness

Drifting temporarily into low consciousness is an inevitable part of life. A body in a state or stress, the presence of strong or persistent low vibrational emotions, symptoms or even tiredness can all have an effect. They key is to allow this to be a temporary state. There are things you can do that will result in you remaining in this low vibrational state or even pull you down further, and there are things you can do to allow yourself to realign and move back into higher consciousness. Whatever state of consciousness we are in our perceptions of life will be impacted. Life could seem rosy or life could seem miserable all depending on whether you are in a low state of consciousness of a high state of consciousness. Knowing that your current perception of yourself and reality often says more about your state of consciousness than the external world can be very useful. Problems ensue when we begin to slip down the spectrum; this impacts how we feel about ourselves which in turn affects how we perceive the world in this moment. These feelings and perceptions influence how we think and act. We generally think that this is "reality" rather than a reflection of our spiraling vibrational state. The tendency is to try and fix the world or fix our feelings, which usually involves more internal thinking keeping us focused on problems as our vibration drops further and our mind gets cluttered. Reality can shift from moment to moment depending on our point of perception and our vibrational state. It is much easier to shift your point of perception and your vibration than it is to shift the world.

When we are aligned we tend to feel good and this, in turn, is reflected in our thinking and behavior. When we feel bad we are more hostile, more agitated, more judgmental and quick to anger. We focus on problems and life seems negative as we spiral down. We think that this is reality rather than just a point of perception. A different reality is just a step away. Trusting that we can naturally float back to our aligned high consciousness space is important. This is not to say that problems or issues don't exist in the world, they do, but addressing them from our high consciousness aligned space is far more useful for us than reacting from low consciousness.

## Moving Back to Higher Consciousness

When you are in a higher state of consciousness, your reality is entirely different. You exhibit compassion, are less reactive, and you flow from your true self. Your focus will be less on what is going wrong and more on finding solutions to make life better. The key to tuning-in is feeling not thinking; the closer you are the more you feel good, in harmony with yourself, and life itself. Your true self is always communicating with you through feelings, intuitions, inner knowing, sparks of insight, and flashes of wisdom. When we are aligned with our true self our vibrational consciousness is high, we feel good, life flows, and we feel connected.

What is important is recognizing where we are on the spectrum. If you don't feel good you know that this will affect your thoughts and perceptions, it doesn't mean that these thoughts and perceptions are real. This is why trying to address a problem or make a decision when you are in a low consciousness space is not a good idea. But trusting that you will gravitate back to being aligned is key. How do you get there? Follow these steps

- Remember that in any moment you can realign with your true self and experience high vibrational consciousness, but not through force or conscious effort.
- Gently encourage yourself to simply *be*; breathe, feel, and allow.
- Stop trying, forcing, or focusing on what is going wrong.
- Remember that all you have to do is be *you* in this moment.
- The only thing that is important is the next thing that you do, so allow yourself to unfold.
- Gently place your attention and intention on what you want, what you wish to experience now, and just get on with what you want to do next.
- Entertain the idea that at the highest level of consciousness all is well, all is well.

## Symptoms as Messengers

When symptoms present themselves—aches, pains, fatigue, stomach upset, even anxiety and depression—what's the first thing that you think about? What's the first thing that you do?

In Western culture our materialistic, reductionist worldview encourages us to view our bodies as machines. The biomedical model views symptoms in a linear fashion arising as a result of injury or the presence of a pathogen. When we have the experience of symptoms our tendency is to assume that something is happening to us; a disease or condition of some sort. We externalize and "pathologize." Of course, this can be deeply relevant when your symptoms do arise as a result of illness or injury. And you'd be right in thinking that the blocked nose and sore throat that you are experiencing on Wednesday is because you "caught" a cold on Monday.

However, when symptoms are not the result of illness or injury, we have to understand them and approach them in a different way. Adopting the usual approach of, "I've got these symptoms this morning because I have fibromyalgia," or "These symptoms are just my anxiety," imposes a level of disempowerment that prevents us from addressing the cause of those symptoms. These statements are saying that the presence of these symptoms are inevitable because I have a condition, a disease. This is biomedical thinking which is not appropriate for chronic medically unexplained symptoms and some "psychological" health problems such as anxiety and depression. Despite our current perspective and interpretation, I believe that intuitively people understand that symptoms are really messengers. They are our body's ways of telling us that something is not right.

As a podcast host and frequent interviewee on radio shows and podcasts, I'm always deeply interested in the lives and experiences of guests and interviewers. In 2015, I had two conversations that were particularly interesting, one with a guest and one as a guest. The first was interviewee Adam Gilbert. Adam is a weight loss expert, life coach, and writer. Before embarking on his journey as a personal weight-loss coach, Adam left college with ambitions of making it big in corporate America. Though, on reflection, the root of these ambitions were not really aligned with Adam's true self. It was more a case that landing a high-paying executive job with good career prospects was the thing to do, what was expected. However, after a reasonably short period of time in the corporate world, he began to experience stomach pain and discomfort that didn't seem to bear any relation to his diet and nutritional intake. The symptoms were sufficiently significant for Adam to step back and look at his life. He knew deep in his core that these symptoms were his body trying to get his attention, trying to get him to do something different. He came to the realization that he was pursuing an executive career for all the wrong reasons—meaning other people's reasons—and that his passions lay elsewhere. He decided what he really wanted to do and then dug deep and found the courage to walk away from corporate life. Almost as soon as he made this decision and took the step of leaving his job his stomach symptoms disappeared without any change in diet or medications.

Arguably Adam was lucky, he had intuitively made the connection between the path his life was taking and the symptoms his body was sending. Donna Gunter didn't make the connection. I was a guest on Donna's *Ultimate Authorities Radio* show talking about the connection between emotions and disease. As I was explaining the Energy-flow principles to her it dawned on her that her symptoms were related to blocked emotion as well. Like Adam, she had been stricken with severe stomach symptoms and had visited her doctor. She told of how her working life had become more stressful as layoffs in the workplace had resulted in an increased workload and increased "stress." Her doctor hadn't asked about her life at work or at home, his focus was on the specific symptoms and what could be done to alleviate them. He conducted a series of tests, which all came back negative, meaning that there were no physical anomalies evident. He referred her to a specialist who started to map out a strategy that involved extensive exploratory surgery to try and identify the problem so it could be solved surgically. A short time after this, and before she was due to go for surgery, Donna left her job. Like Adam, her symptoms vanished almost overnight. Initially, she was relieved because these debilitating symptoms were no longer present and it meant she didn't need expensive surgery. However, on reflection, it concerned her that her doctor hadn't even considered that the stress and emotion in her life could be the underlying cause of the symptoms she was experiencing, and so addressing these was never an option.

One important point I need to emphasize is that I am not advocating making major life decisions in order to get away from symptoms. In these examples, it just happens that walking away from jobs that were not right for the individuals concerned resulted in an alleviation of symptoms. However, such drastic action is rarely needed and should only be considered as a last resort. The key lesson in these cases is that we need to recognize that when our body produces symptoms it is trying to get our attention. The symptoms are trying to alert us to the fact that something is wrong.

Intuitively we know this, just as Adam Gilbert knew. However, when symptoms become severe or chronic, as in Donna's case, we stop trusting ourselves, in fact, we stop asking ourselves. We align ourselves with the Western materialistic mechanistic perspective of the body, assuming that something is happening to us and we need something outside of ourselves. I'm not suggesting that we always know what is wrong with us, but I am suggesting that we can attune to ourselves and trust our intuition. Knowing that when we are experiencing symptoms of a health challenge our body is trying to get our attention; it is seeking to convey a message to us.

I'm sure you've heard stories of people who sensed there was something wrong only to be told by their doctor that no evidence of a health challenge. Then at some point later problems were uncovered, diagnoses were given, and in some instances these were too late to halt the advance of terminal disease. We need a balance of internal trust alongside external knowledge. I think that it is vitally important that we consult with medical professionals and I would never advocate abandoning medicine even if the biomedical model exhibits some limitations. However, this does not need to be an either-or model and trusting our own intuition is also vital. This leads us on to our next key principle:

## True Empowerment: Inside-Out Living

Empowerment is a word that is frequently used in the world of health, personal development and business; maybe too frequently because its meaning seems to have been diluted to such an extent that its meaning and interpretation varies enormously. The Collins English dictionary defines empowerment as: "having qualities that give a person or a group of people the means to take more control of their lives and become stronger and more independent." Empowerment from an Energy-flow perspective is not about control or power, rather it is about awareness and responsibility and what you create in your life. Responsibility is not control; we can take responsibility for our emotions and the actions we take, but we cannot control our emotions. We can take responsibility for what we do with the thoughts in our heads but we cannot control the thoughts themselves. In truth, we are never really in control and we are certainly not in control of external events. But crucially we don't need to be in control. If you have ever felt insecure or overwhelmed there is a very good chance that you will have tried to control your life circumstances or the people in your life. There seems to be an unconscious drive that if we are not in control of how we feel internally we need to control external circumstances. The reason we tend to do this is because unconsciously we believe that external events directly cause how we feel and because we have a strong drive to escape our emotional discomfort and feel good, we fixate on controlling external events.

We're all familiar with the notion of, "I'll be happy when . . ." If you fill in the blank it could be, "I'll be happy when I get the job promotion," or "I'll be happy when the kids are back in school," or "I'll be happy when I retire," and so on. At one level you may think that these statements are merely figures of speech, ways of talking that don't really have any deeper meaning. However, they do have a deeper meaning, in that they will impact your perceptions of life and the way you think and behave. They are representations of the belief that what happens "out there" causes what I feel "in here." This makes it all about the events, something external to us; external and uncontrollable. The flip side of this is that I become a victim of circumstance; my feelings are completely dependent on external circumstances. These circumstances could be the behavior, words, and actions of others or simply life events. When this happens we may find ourselves saying things like, "He made me angry," or "She always makes me frustrated." Again with these statements we are reinforcing the deep belief that how we feel is completely dictated and controlled by external events.

However, have you noticed that there are times when something can happen and the feelings you have today are different from the feelings you had last week or even yesterday? This could be something that someone says or does that last week seemed to "make" you frustrated, while this week it seemed to go over your head. What does this mean? Could it be that how we feel is not directly controlled by external circumstances?

As we discussed in the previous chapter, our feelings arise from a complex interplay of a number of factors and primarily come from inside us. Taking responsibility for these feelings and what we do that follows them is the essence of empowerment. Assuming other people are responsible for how we feel and for what happens to us is giving away our responsibility, which is disempowering. We also know that our state of consciousness and level of alignment with our true self will impact how we perceive life events and ourselves. The more we develop our awareness of our feelings and emotions the more we can take responsibility for them and become empowered.

There is a school of thought that we need to transcend our emotion or control it in some way in order to achieve peace of mind or enlightenment. The simple response to this is that we don't and we can't. If you are remotely familiar with the world of new age spirituality or even personal development, you'll have come across the idea that our goal is not to experience "negative" emotions anymore, and by altering our thinking patterns we can transcend them. I went through a period in the early 2000s, whereby for some reason I was attracting a large number of Buddhist clients. I recognize that there are many ways of interpreting religions and ideologies and the Buddhists that I was seeing were entertaining the notion that negative emotions such as anger were not to be experienced. Now I don't know whether this was because emotions were thought to be the output of the mind, or whether it was believed that thinking or the mind could manipulate emotional experience. Either way, negative emotions were to be transcended and they were only to feel joy and compassion. What they didn't realize was that their intelligent body produced anger, even if they didn't think it did. So in effect, their egoic-mind had made a decision about what they should experience. Rather than recognizing that acceptance involves allowing everything that the intelligent body sends they had decided that emotions came from the egoic-mind and therefore could be controlled by the mind. The denial of anger and other such emotions led to suppression and the result was a tap on the shoulder in the form of symptoms.

The other issue is control. As a thinking and mind-centered society, we have the notion that we can control everything. This probably goes back to the idea that man has dominion over the earth and all that roams across it. If we can control the earth and the animals we should be able to control ourselves. But in truth we don't have control, and in seeking to attain control we move further and further into egoic-mind and away from the flow of the true self, the intelligent body and the energy flow of life. When we transcend the controlling mind we can begin to see that we don't have control over how we feel and we don't need to control how we feel. As we begin to become more empowered and responsible for ourselves we experience more of an Energy-flow and release the need to control people and the environment outside ourselves.

There is a very definite energy or frequency to disempowerment, which is quite different from the vibration of empowerment. When we are empowered we experience our Energy-flow and are aligned with our core frequency. This means we feel connected and derive the other "benefits" from residing towards the higher vibrational end of our consciousness spectrum. When we give away our power and act as if someone else is responsible for how we feel, we tend to feel misaligned, shaky, vulnerable, and excessively emotional, and we slip down the consciousness spectrum. These feelings can really come to the fore when talking about our situation. For example, if I tell you how Mike Williams makes me angry by the things he does and there's nothing I can do about it, negative feelings will arise, and I'll mistakenly believe that these feelings are present because what I am describing is true. However, I would like you to entertain a different perspective. In our chapter on emotion I talked about how negative feelings were feedback indicating that we needed to align with our true self, they are a tap on the shoulder encouraging us to act authentically in this moment. So the uncomfortable feelings we are experiencing when describing our disempowered state are arising because we are deviating from who we are, from our true self. As we slip down the vibrational spectrum more negative feelings arise. We are allowing ourselves to become misaligned. Our true nature is empowered, almost as if our true self knows that we are responsible for ourselves and when we give responsibility to others it has to somehow get our attention to let us know we are living a lie. I have had this experience many times where the words out of my mouth did not align with my inner truth and the result was uncomfortable feelings. Those negative feelings can be quite intense and then recede incredibly quickly when stepping back into an empowered space and taking responsibility for feelings rather than attributing them to something or someone else.

We cannot extricate or separate ourselves from our environment, and as such we are always going to have feelings that appear to correlate with external events; however, by recognizing the role we play in creating our experience and by taking responsibility for our own emotions we become empowered. As we become empowered we are better placed to look inside ourselves for guidance rather than assuming that all the answers lie outside of ourselves. This leads us to our next foundational notion.

## Beyond Dualism

How often do you find yourself talking or thinking about something being good or bad, right or wrong, should or shouldn't? These are examples of dualistic thinking and they are so common they tend to dominate almost every aspect of our thinking and perception. The notion of duality or polarity is so prevalent that it seems almost hardwired into the human brain.

There is a level of dualistic thinking that seems pretty obvious on the face of it. We are all guilty of presenting choices such as good or bad, right or wrong, black or white. However, what is particularly interesting is that the scope of dualistic thinking goes way beyond the obvious examples of good and bad or right and wrong. It tends to be the case that when making decisions about anything in life people tend to give themselves two options. This can often mean I either do it or I don't do it; or, I can do it this way or that way. Each time the tendency is to entertain the possibility of two choices. It seems almost bizarre that we would restrict ourselves in such a manner, reducing our own choices and options, cutting down on potentials and possibilities.

When I first really noticed this, I would be telling my clients and then give them 2 options on how we would move forward. It was so ingrained in me that even when talking the talk I wasn't walking the walk. So why is dualistic thinking a problem? Well, it's not so much that it is a problem, rather that it is constricting. Moving into an Energy-flow is about expansion and opportunity. When we constrict ourselves we limit ourselves, we remove possibility, options, and opportunity.

The second point about dualistic thinking is that it requires judgment. Every time one option is selected over another a judgment is made. This largely goes against the wisdom of our intuition and selecting one option over another can, therefore, feel somewhat uncomfortable in the body. When we can open our minds and think in quantum terms of everything being connected, the idea of two separate poles existing in isolation dissolves as we can begin to step back and see the bigger picture of connection and holism. As we do this we can reflect on greater potentials, more options, opportunities and outcomes. Transcending duality in everyday life can have an enormous impact on our sense of freedom, which facilitates alignment with our core frequency If you would like to play with expanding dualism in your everyday life, try this.

1. For two days have your focus on where your thinking and speaking is dualistic—where you are presenting two choices to yourself, or talking about right/wrong, good/ bad, should/shouldn't, etc.

2. Stop, breathe and change your words and your thoughts—imagine stepping away from the duality paradigm to entertain a broader perspective or spectrum of choices and ideas. Notice how your experience changes as a broader spectrum and choices are entertained.

3. Follow through with actions to support your new way of seeing the situation—this helps if you can recognize you have been constricting yourself with dualities, whereas opening up to more possibilities gives you a new sense of freedom. As duality tends to present itself in little ways in our everyday life, I would suggest starting with small, seemingly trivial changes so you can get used to the concept and its implementation.

## Riding the Wave of Homeostasis

If you were to fall and graze your knee you know a process will take place whereby your blood will coagulate, a scab will form over the graze, then new skin will be formed underneath the scab. Bit by bit the scab will fall from your knee as the healing process runs its course. The same process takes place if you were to have a few too many glasses of wine at dinner. You could wake up the following day feeling a little groggy with a headache and nausea. However, with absolutely no intervention within a few hours you should feel normal again. These are very simple examples of the self-correcting nature of homeostasis that works throughout our mind-body system. It's as if our bodies have a blueprint or template for health and wellness and if we get out of the way we can allow this process to take place. The exact same thing will happen with our emotional state. This is most evident in children. Children can be sad or angry one minute then happy and laughing the next. They don't hold grudges; they allow the natural flow of emotional energy to take place and they self-correct back to their default state.

When we think about improving our health, vitality, happiness and fulfillment, there can be a tendency to look outside of ourselves assuming we need to do something or get something in order to feel as we want to feel. However, as human beings, we have immense capacity to heal on every level and unleash and fulfil our own potentials without relying on regimes, techniques or structures. In fact, our natural default mode, our template, is to be in an Energy-flow, aligned with our true self and in doing so experience health and wellness.

Let me clarify what I mean when I talk about regimes and techniques. I'm not suggesting that doing a technique is necessarily a bad thing if intuitively you are drawn to it. However, there is a difference between being intuitively drawn to something as opposed to thinking that you should or have to do something. Without doubt you will have had the experience of thinking there is something you should do. A frequent question that I am asked is, "Should I meditate?," to which I quickly reply "No." Believing that we need to, or should do something in order to complete ourselves, or be healthy is simply not helpful. A better starting position is to be truly empowered and recognize you have all the resources you need internally and that immediately seeking external intervention is not the best idea. Sometimes it can be useful to address the question of why, when thinking about doing some technique or applying some tool. For the most part, the answer lies will be because it just hadn't occurred to us that we have the capacity, ability, aptitude, and resources ourselves without having to reach for something off the shelf.

There is also the issue that through our biofield we are naturally connected to everything in life, so what goes on outside us is not completely separate and distinct from what is inside us. We are a microcosm of the entire universe. Inside and outside us are in a continual flux of influencing and being influenced; there exists the potential for simultaneous creation both inside you and outside you. This means that aligning with the internal wisdom that is your true self will foster the best solutions whether you are guided to create and uncover internally or externally.

There will be instances, especially in relation to health, where the problem may be so severe that the body's ability to self-correct is unable to function properly. When we have a cut our body heals itself as long as the conditions allow the body to do so. What we know is that if your knee doesn't stop bleeding or if your hangover doesn't go, there is a problem, there is something preventing the natural process of homeostasis. In the example of our cut, in some cases the cut may be so deep and wide that that stitches are needed. Of course, the stitches don't do the healing, the stitches merely facilitate an environment that allows the body to do the work of healing itself. So sometimes the body needs a nudge in the right direction, when it has this nudge and the environment allows it, healing takes place.

However, too much or incorrect external intervention can destabilize the self-correcting healing process. How do we know if this is the case? If a problem persists, there is a very good chance that the attempted solution we are implementing is holding the problem in place. This idea is described in Paul Watzlawick's brilliant book, *Change: Principles of Problem Formation and Problem Resolution*. In this book, Watzlawick describes First Order and Second Order Change in the process of solving a problem. First order change describes the process whereby we implement a solution that works in direct opposition to the problem. An example could be that when you feel cold you put additional layers of clothing on, like a woolen jumper, to help increase the temperature of your body. You feel warmer, the problem has been solved, this is a successful intervention.

Imagine for a moment being in a revolving door that you are not able to see through. You begin to push and the door starts moving, then it stops and you are partway round. What do you do? You push harder, don't you? It's the obvious solution. But what if the door won't move, it feels jammed? Do you push even harder? Most people would, it seems obvious. But how long do you push before you decide that this attempted solution isn't working? What if you knew that someone on the other side of your revolving door was experiencing the exact same problem as you, they are pushing just as hard as you are pushing and the harder you push the harder they push. With this additional information you realize that your attempted solution of pushing harder is keeping the problem in place. This is where Watzlawick's Second Order Change comes into play. When the problem persists we need to turn our attention to the attempted solution we are implementing and change that. In our simple example of the revolving door, if we stop pushing and the person on the other side continues pushing the door moves. Even though it is not moving in the direction we originally intended, by turning around and walking in the opposite direction we can move through the door and into the building.

The same is true for our emotional healing. Earlier in the chapter I mentioned Weebles (the toys) and their ability to wobble and then return to their natural default upright position. When we experience a low vibrational negative emotion, it's a bit like a Weeble taking a knock and starting to wobble. If we allow ourselves to feel and process that emotion we can stay aligned with our true self and after a bit of wobbling back and forth we return to our neutral position reasonably quickly. However, what often happens is we start thinking in order to solve or resolve our emotion, or to find meaning in it and this has the effect of keeping the feeble wobbling at a faster and faster pace. As this happens we drop down our vibrational spectrum from high consciousness to low consciousness and in doing so we being misaligned and out of touch with our true self.

So what are we learning for all this? First, we need to trust our own inner ability to self-heal and self-correct. As we are evolving, our tendency is to gravitate towards high vibrational consciousness, this is happening naturally. When we get off track and face problems we either need to allow ourselves to naturally self-correct or we need a simple nudge. If our problem persists there is a good chance that we have lost faith in our own ability to self-correct and we are seeking an external solution or solutions and these solutions are holding the problem in place. The biggest example of this for sufferers of chronic fatigue and pain conditions is when an attempted solution is to rest and stop engaging in life, because it appears that these cause symptoms. However, just like pushing the revolving door harder, these attempted solutions hold the problem in place. To experience health we have to align with our true self, this means we have to be unleashed to experience ourselves fully. Curtailing life because of symptoms ultimately results in a massive buildup of frustration from our intelligent body in an attempt to have us align with our true self's desire for self expression and freedom.

## Open Awareness

Open Awareness is a simple principle, it invites you to step back and open up. If you imagine expanding all of your senses and merging them as they flow like a field or wave that gently undulates beyond the physical boundaries of your body. This open awareness emerges from consciousness, which is almost like emerging from nothing, just potential.

In Western society, critical thinking and reasoning are viewed as the pinnacle of human ability. Using our bulbous cerebral cortex to navigate our way through every problem, it is almost instinctive in Western society to use focused thinking as the sole medium through which we experience life. I'd like to be clear at this stage what I mean by the words thinking and thought, because I'm conscious that, just like the words emotion and stress, people have their own ideas about words mean. I am also conscious that different ideas and models use the word thought to mean anything from unconscious cognitive processes to a field of energy that exists beyond the boundaries of the physical body. For our purposes, I'm going to define thinking as a conscious process or white noise that may be taking place just outside of conscious awareness. What I mean by white noise is a buzz or blur that you may be aware of more than specific words. Conscious thought could be defined as internal dialogue, sounds and pictures in your head. The white noise is something that if you were to stop for a moment you might detect. You could think of it as looking carefully into a smoky room and with a light squint you can make out what is going on in that room. The white noise in your head just outside of your awareness is the same. Thoughts that are droning on.

I don't consider that every cognitive process, including memory, attention, unconscious evaluations, appraisals and beliefs, are thinking or thought. So we will define thinking as something going on in your head that you are pretty much aware of. I am also going to suggest that focus is more aligned with thinking and thought, where as Open Awareness is not. If you were to take a magnifying glass outside on a bright sunny day and align it with the rays of light cascading from the sun, you could focus the energy of the sun into a single concentrated beam. Focus is a narrowing of attention and energy where as open awareness is a dispersing of attention; a widening expansion that takes you away from thought.

As you're reading this page now, let me invite you to soften and expand. Open your awareness and feel all your senses merge and drift beyond the physical boundaries of your body. Avoid focusing on any one thing; simply allow your awareness to be present and expand. Without thought you can hold an intention of aligning with your true self, and allowing homeostasis to run its course, you might find that your breathing becomes a little slower, a little deeper, and more regular; in fact you will probably feel more aligned. You may find that your attention is momentarily pulled from different areas, maybe something comes into your visual field, then you feel something move in your right leg. With Open Awareness you can observe these happenings without comment, without judgment and without question.

## From Resistance to Allowing

If you spend enough time on Facebook, you'll probably get to see a picture with a quote from Carl Jung saying, "What you resist, persists." Jung was referring to aspects of ourselves that we resist. The notion came from his work relating to what he called our "shadow" selves; those aspects of us that we prefer to keep hidden or that remain outside of our conscious awareness. Jung suggested that the more we resist those aspects of ourselves that maybe we don't like the more fractured we become and the more problems we experience.

The notion that it is resistance, both internal and external, that causes suffering is an idea that can be traced back to Buddhist and Taoist philosophy. There's absolutely no doubt that resistance is a critical factor in our ride through life. But the interesting bit is that resistance is insidious, it sneaks in the back door. We're resisting without knowing we're resisting. We're pushing away, tensing up, blocking every day and we just don't realize we're doing it.

So as you review your day to day experience now, you could be thinking, "Well, I get up in the morning, take a shower, get the kids ready for school, then I get ready for work and head out the door. I do a day at the office, come home, get dinner ready, yadda yadda yadda, . . . I don't see how I'm resisting or what I'm resisting." That's a fair point, and exactly my point. As you go through those simple everyday activities that make up your current experience of life, you are unlikely to notice the role that resistance plays. Let's have a little look in more detail at what resistance is and what it entails, then we'll move on to looking at the opposite of resistance, which is allowance.

Let's start by keeping it simple. Our experience of life comprises the external—what goes on outside of us; and the internal—what takes place inside us. And, as we know there is an interplay and connected flow between the two. Unsurprisingly, we have the capacity and tendency to resist both. What that means is that we often resist what happens in life and then we resist how we feel. Sometimes we are doing this at the same time, and other times not.

If we start by looking at resisting the external, how do we actually do that? It often starts with expectations; we have ideas about how we want things to be. I'm not necessarily talking about long-term big life goals, I'm talking about little everyday events. We want to get to work on time; we expect to be able to buy the food we want when we go food shopping; we expect the water to run when we turn the shower on in the morning. For the most part, our lives consist of a series of moments woven together with simple activities juxtaposing themselves into those moments.

When my eldest daughter was about 18 months old, she seemed to find herself entering the dreaded "terrible twos," a time when kids begin to have tantrums. Parents know that the tantrums that kids have at this age are very different from when they are upset about something. The tantrum is an experience that seems to take complete control and there is nothing really parents can do at this age, aside from enduring the tantrums. I had gone through a two-week period where I was feeling significant surges of anger inside around the time my daughter was experiencing tantrums. I wasn't outwardly expressing this anger, but I was both curious and concerned about the level of anger I was experiencing internally.

I sat down one Sunday night with my wife and told her what I was experiencing and that I really needed to understand what was going on with me. The following morning, I was getting my daughter dressed on the landing just outside our bedroom. As we hit the halfway stage of the process the tantrum genie blessed us and my daughter exploded into shrieks and wails. Almost immediately I felt this huge surge of anger. Determined to get to the bottom of my experience, I went and sat on my bed to practice some open awareness. I do possess the ability to be able to observe my experience, and what I noticed was my head saying, "Why can't you just get dressed, why do you have to play up like this." I was then able to pull my attention down into my body and feel the physical sensations of the emotion. As I did, my head went quiet and the amount of emotion I was feeling dropped dramatically. My attention went back up into my head and the same words started to appear again, so I dropped my attention once again into my body to feel. This was fascinating, if I were to give you a rating out of ten for the severity of my emotional experience, when my attention was in my head the amount of anger and frustration felt to me like an 8/10. When I dropped my attention into my body and allowed myself to just feel the physical sensations of the emotion, the amount of emotion I was feeling dropped to about a three.

What was going on? The language in my head was an example of resistance. With just two sentences I was resisting the fact that my daughter was experiencing a tantrum. When I brought my attention into my body, I was allowing my daughter to have her tantrum without resistance and I was allowing myself to experience emotion. The result was a drop from 8/10 to 3/10.

Having realized that all I needed to do was allow, I felt what to do next. I knew that I couldn't stop my daughter's tantrum and that she would calm down within a minute or two, so I allowed myself to experience my frustration and I got dressed. Within two minutes her tantrum subsided as did my frustration. This was a major eureka moment. I'd known that when the head involved itself in emotion, the experience of emotion usually got worse, but I hadn't realized that by resisting, it more than doubled the negative experience.

Resistance of external events and situations isn't always going to be an experience where we are aware of our head obviously resisting. Sometimes you might just feel tension in your body. However, when you bring your attention onto that tension, you will be aware that either consciously or unconsciously you are resisting what is happening, you probably have an expectation.

Resisting internal feelings follows the same pattern. There is usually a tension as we try to push away what we are feeling, or there will be some internal dialogue, along the lines of, "I don't want to feel this," or "I don't want to be the kind of person that feels this." The latter probably being the most common. We so frequently attach meaning to our feelings that we see them as a representation of us, who we are. Feelings are just feelings, and what we feel this week could potentially change and be different next week. Either way, attaching meaning to feelings usually results in us resisting those feelings, which in turn results in them either getting stuck or getting amplified.

It's hardly surprising that we resist our internal feelings. It appears that the areas of the brain activated during the experience of physical pain are the same areas activated when we experience emotional pain—this is probably why we talk about emotional pain. As humans our desire is to move away from discomfort towards comfort is instinctive, so there's little surprise that we want to escape our uncomfortable feelings.

The irony, of course, is that resistance of both the external and the internal exacerbates our negative experience. What's bizarre is that it seems so instinctive to resist. We do the same with physical pain, as we wince, tense up and hold our breath. The key to easing our experience is allowance.

Allowing doesn't mean being happy about what's going on or how we are feeling. Allowing simply means observing. In truth by allowing you are being flexible. If I leave my clinic after a busy day and find that there is an empty space where my car had previously been, the fact that my car has been stolen is going to hit me like a punch in the stomach. My head will want to take this emotion and run with it, like Usain Bolt in full flight. It'll want to say things like, "What the f**k, I can't believe it, this can't be happening, it can't be happening to me now." If I let my head do that the amount of emotion I'm experiencing will double or even triple. With such a significant event, there's a strong possibility that a huge amount of emotion will affect my cognitive processing to such a degree that it'll render me incapable of doing anything. If this were to happen, I'd be rooted to the spot, spiraling down the consciousness spectrum. If you're ever walking down the street and you see someone rooted to the spot simply staring at a parking space there's a good chance their car used to be there.

If I allow what has happened, and I allow myself to feel the hurt, anger and frustration I will be able to direct my attention to what I do next given the situation is as it is. I then quickly reach for my mobile phone and call my wife, the police and the insurance company. The hurt and anger aren't going away quickly and as long as they are there the temptation to get into my head and resist will be lurking in the background, waiting to pounce. However, as I start to take productive, constructive action there is the possibility that the emotional landscape of my mind and body will begin to change. If, however, I get caught in my head and fail to take constructive action the negativity will spiral and I'll get caught in a vortex of negativity, like a whirlwind. There's a good chance that I will regurgitate my internal experience as I talk to friends, all the while strengthening the pattern and making it a habit. Have you ever noticed yourself in this pattern, where you resist some events or circumstances because they "shouldn't" have happened? You tell friends and family and they reinforce your experience and validate your experience. This is when you get stuck in what we're going to call the "victim-vortex," a low consciousness energy spiral that keeps you out of alignment with your true self.

> Mary was a government employee and worked in a large office with. She had a close group of four friends at work and they all shared the office. They reported to different managers and performed different jobs so there was always plenty to talk about at coffee break, lunch and after work. Mary's boss was pretty disgruntled at work and had a tendency to take this out on his small team of six, but for some reason it was Mary who always seemed to get the worst of it. In fact, when she thought about it, she couldn't remember the last time that any of the others in the team experienced the same "treatment" as she did. Fatigue, headaches, and low level depression were frequently part of Mary's life experience, and the symptoms seemed to be increasing in duration and intensity. Most days she would experience some interaction with her boss that would either leave her with increases in her symptoms or some level or body tension. Like most people, Mary thought life was life; it's something that just happens and you roll with it. As we started to look at her experience a pattern emerged of resistance to external events without taking constructive action; resistance to her feelings (because she didn't want to be the type of person who was "upset by a jerk").

So how can we begin to take that seemingly giant step from resisting to allowing? As I've already said, allowing doesn't mean being happy about what's happening, it simply means acknowledging what the situation or circumstances are presenting and allowing the energy to flow. The resistance often starts in the mind with something like, "Why is this happening, I hate it when this happens." As soon as we utter words to this effect to ourselves in our mind, the intensity of emotion experienced amplifies dramatically—emotions kick in and take over. We often think that these emotions are created in response to the event, situation or person. They are not; the event, situation or person has your intelligent body producing a small amount of emotion, just enough to give you a tap on the shoulder. The mind takes over and makes it enormous. This exercise is something to play with if you would like to experience more allowing and less resistance in everyday life.

1. Stop for a moment and think about something you don't like or would prefer not to happen. This could be something very small and seemingly trivial.
2. As you think about it notice what you feel in the body and where you feel it. The chances are you are experiencing a tightness or tension somewhere in your body.
3. This might be accompanied by some mental chatter along the lines of, "I hate it when this happens," "Why can't it just be like . . ."; "Oh, no"; "Oh why?" and other such mental comments.
4. Bring your attention into your body in order to reduce the metal chatter; focus on the physical sensations you are experiencing.
5. Feel into the notion that, "Given this (the circumstances or situation) is as it is, what do I want to do about it or what can I do; what do I want instead of what's happening; what do I wish to experience." From there, take some action if you can.
6. Now that you have consciously acknowledged and learned what resistance feels like allow yourself to begin to notice when these sensations arise in your daily life. Resistance will usually manifest in tensions somewhere in the body, this could be the forehead, the chest, the shoulders, arms, legs, or stomach. As you learn to pay attention you will feel where resistance manifests itself physically in your body.
7. When the physical sensations arise, stop, breathe and

allow yourself to feel the emotions associated with the situation or event.

8. Accept and allow the event or situation to exist, then decide what you want to do and wish to experience given that this event or situation does exist.

9. Make this your focus for at least one week, then revisit it as often as needed to fully embed it into your life.

For the Bigger Picture of Life

1. Acknowledge and accept everything that is happening in your life, both specific situations and the bigger picture. Stop for a moment and reflect on this. Think about your current life and where you feel resistance.

2. Acknowledge and accept everything you feel, both comfortable and uncomfortable feelings.

3. Bring your attention into your body, breathe, then acknowledge the events or circumstances and feel into your options of what you wish to experience next. What do you want to happen instead of what is happening?

4. Remember you have the potential to create your experience, so allow yourself to move in alignment with your deepest feelings and wishes in the moment.

## How to Really Step Up: Live Like You Mean It

If you were to stop for a moment and look at your everyday life, do you find that you feel almost trapped in a cycle, almost like a hamster on a wheel? Do you feel you are directing your life, or do you feel your life is running you? As I look around the pace of life is on the increase, time is literally speeding up leaving us feeling that we have more to do and less time to do it in. A frantic energy grips us as we struggle to pay the bills, meet deadlines, and get everything done; all the chores of life. If you are like the majority, you are stuck in a cycle of debt, with mortgages, overdrafts, and loans keeping you in a perpetual state of mild to major worry.

The impact of all this can keep us stuck in the negative spiral of survival, ever so slightly out of alignment with our core frequency. Your outlook is likely to be one of coping, not really fully engaging with life, doing what you need to do to get through each day. At its very worst this spiral of survival can result in a chronic expectation of negativity; expecting things to go wrong, rueing missed opportunities, complaining about what's not working and what's not happening—continually resisting.

This negative spiral keeps us trapped in a vortex of negativity that saps our energy, leads to excessive worry and confusion and impacts upon the quality of our life and what we experience in day-to-day life. Like a vortex or whirlwind, once we get stuck in this energetic pattern it can be very difficult to see a way out, and we can spiral down and down.

This trance-like way of living, simply existing, can sneak up on us. One day we're loving life, making conscious choices, moving forward and the next we seem to be observers of our life, as if somehow someone else grabbed the steering wheel and stuck us in the trunk. Of course it doesn't have to be like that, even when it seems that life is moving on without you, or running its course leaving you on the sidelines, you are only a step away from re-engaging with your life, stepping-up and living like you really mean it, like you really want to ring the most out of every single moment on earth.

If you have ever read anything about research conducted on those who have experienced near-death experiences, or NDEs. There are overwhelming similarities in what takes place during the NDEs, but crucially and overwhelmingly, those that have been through this change their lives. They see this as an opportunity to begin living, really living without compromise, without excuses; an attitude of taking life by the scruff of the neck.

What's important for us is the understanding that this is much more than approach and attitude. What results in a change of interaction with life, more of an alignment with true self and this in turn impacts our ongoing emotional experience of life. The idea that simply changing one's mind or thinking different thoughts will change everything is flawed. A shift in attitude is only useful if it precipitates a change in behavior that sees an alignment with true self and the resulting behavioral change and emotional experience. In the absence of these thoughts are useless. You can think all the positive thoughts you like, but if you fail to align with your true self and shift the way you interact with life, your emotional experience is unlikely to significantly change, and it's all about the emotion not the thinking. In fact, trying to think positive thoughts is not the best option either, because will keep you locked in your head and out of touch with your true self.

## Let's Play Offense, Not Defense

Okay, so I'm borrowing from American football terminology with this section, but as we begin to go through this principle you'll understand why. In life we move towards pleasure and away from discomfort and pain, it's a simple survival mechanism that can be overridden, but can persist unchecked if we allow it.

> Some years ago I was working with a client who had been suffer-ing with chronic fatigue syndrome for a number of years. Lucy was in her late twenties and had a young son. She lived sev-eral hundred miles away from me, so our sessions were a mix of phone and face-to-face when she took the plunge and asked her mother to drive her across country. Much to my, and her mother's delight, Lucy responded well to working with me and experienced a dramatic reduction in symptoms over a period of months. We decided to have a gap of three months between ses-sions to give her a chance to get on with her life and put every-thing she had learned into practice on a consistent basis.
>
> When I called Lucy for her appointment, I was greeted by a wispy and frail voice, "Thank God, it's you," she said, "I've had so many symptoms back this week I had to go to the doctor." Over the course of the next ten minutes, Lucy described what had happened. Five days prior to our session she experienced some very minor symptoms, but, as is often the case, one of those symptoms was something she had not experienced since the very early days of the CFS. This mild pain in her right shoulder sent her into a state of fear. She told me that the last time this symptom had presented itself it had moved quickly throughout her body. This time, rather than going through our process and identifying the cause of the symptom, Lucy went into defensive mode. She slipped back into fear and started looking at how to manage her life to avoid symptoms. She went straight back into the "illness lifestyle" that she had adopted when debilitated

*with CFS. The more she had sought to avoid symptoms and life, the more the symptoms spread. The pain moved from her right shoulder right throughout her chest and stomach. Her chest was so tight she was having difficulties breathing. On the morning of our appointment she had been to see her GP to see if he could do something about her breathing difficulties. He told her that he couldn't detect anything wrong with her heart or lungs and told her to rest and come back in a few days.*

*After she told me what had happened I reminded her of everything she knew. We talked about everything she had done to alleviate her symptoms by putting the process and principles into action. Within about 30 minutes she recognized what had triggered the symptom episode to begin with and she could see exactly how she had changed from being focused on living life to the full to receding completely back into an illness lifestyle pattern. By the time we ended the call the symptoms had all but gone and she was breathing clearly again.*

Does this mean the symptoms were all in her head? Absolutely not. What it shows is the power of emotion, particularly fear and how this can impact behavior and ongoing emotions. It wasn't just the fear that caused this acceleration of symptoms over the course of five days, it was the fact that the fear impacted her ongoing interaction with life. She stopped living, she moved into defensive mode and this lead to a whole series of emotions. Remember that our emotions are providing feedback about our ongoing interaction with the environment. An emotion you experience right now might impact your behavior for the coming minutes, even hours or days. When these emotions buildup in the stress bucket their toxicity leads to overflow and symptoms.

Lucy had given us the perfect example of the defensive play.

## The Defensive Play

As symptoms increase, the focus is on getting away from the symptoms to minimize their impact. While this seems like the most logical option, it can be more of a running away from symptoms rather than trying to understand what they are trying to say. This usually stems from fear and frustration; fear because the origin of symptoms may not be clear and their progression in this moment remains unknown; frustration because having symptoms in that moment may curtail the current activity and have a negative impact on life.

The attempted solutions are usually to want to rest or to escape from how you are feeling, in order to reduce symptoms or manage symptoms. This option rarely leads to the complete cessation of symptoms in the short term and never results in a complete elimination of symptoms or "cure" in the longer term.

Over time the defensive play results in an "illness lifestyle," this is a life that is markedly different from the sort of life you would be leading in the absence of symptoms. The danger with the illness lifestyle is the insidious nature with which it creeps up on you. Small changes here and there, avoiding certain activities or people builds up over time, until your entire life has been turned on its head and completely revolves around having symptoms or avoiding symptoms. It seems absolutely inevitable at some level as doctors may be telling you to rest and the only discernible pattern that accompanies symptoms is doing too much or eating certain foods.

However, the defensive play is not our friend. In the short term, it distracts us from finding the true cause of symptoms in the moment and in the longer term it shackles us and renders us incapable of living a normal life.

### The Offensive Play

Throughout this book the principles and practices that will be offered are based on stepping into the offensive mode, the offensive play. The key principle that underpins the offensive play is that our goal is not to escape symptoms, our goal is to experience freedom, personal freedom. To live a life in alignment with our true self, to be the full expression of ourselves. This takes the focus away from symptoms and onto living a life that is in alignment with who we are and what we want. This doesn't mean ignoring symptoms, in fact quite the opposite. It is important that we pay attention to symptoms because they are offering important feedback and communication. However, there is a massive difference between being aware of symptoms in order to act on their communications and altering our lives in because we feel shackled by symptoms.

The Energy-flow model offers an explanation for a primary cause of symptoms, so understanding why symptoms are there helps us to take the appropriate action to act on that cause. This proactive action is not about trying to minimize or escape symptoms, it's about acting on the cause and then focusing on moving towards what you want right now, what you wish to experience right now. Knowing that you will be far better served by adopting the offensive play at the outset serves as a good foundation for making progress towards optimum health.

## Developing Self-Trust

Trust is the ability to depend upon; it is an assured reliance on truth and ability, it is something on which confidence is placed. I am inviting you to trust yourself. Your true self always offers you truth in the form of the communication it sends and it has the ability to effectively direct you through life. Self-trust is simply acting in alignment with your deeper intuitive feelings without being talked out of it by your thinking chattering egoic-mind, the part of you that churns out the effects of conditioning and programming and tries to have to believe and act as if you are not worthy or good enough to be trusted.

Developing self-trust requires you are inward looking, internally referenced rather than externally referenced. As I look at my children grow I can see there is an interesting mix of a developing brain that becomes increasingly self-aware and sees itself as separate from others, coupled with a society and educational system that encourages constant comparisons. Reflecting and comparing are examples of being externally referenced.

Traditionally self-esteem and developing self-esteem is seen in the same light, we are encouraged to view ourselves in relation to others. Our attention is drawn externally rather than internally. The result is that we judge ourselves and we do this in relation to others and external standards. When this gets to the extreme our focus is completely fixated on external ideals and standards and we lose connection to who we are and what is right for us.

| TRADITIONAL SELF CONFIDENCE | ENERGY-FLOW TRUE SELF CONFIDENCE |
|---|---|
| Outward-looking | Inward-looking |
| Comparing self with others | Flowing authentically without comparison |
| Wanting to fit in, to "normalize" | Striving for individual expression |
| Seeking external validation | Internal validation through trust and feeling |
| Conditional | Unconditional |
| Dependent on skills and knowledge | Dependent only on standing in your own truth |

*Timothy was a junior competitive cyclist, he first came to see me at age 12, suffering from a high level of anxiety. His symptoms had progressed to the level that he was no longer cycling and was experiencing increasingly severe anxiety at school. When we first started working together our goal was to reduce the anxiety symptoms, we didn't even think about cycling and getting back to competitive racing.*

*Cycling was Timothy's love and not being able to cycle at his club with his teammates was in itself having an exacerbating impact on the anxiety that was presenting itself. It became clear pretty early on that Timothy was almost completely externally referenced. This began with a desire to impress his coach and make his parents happy, as he saw it—even though it made little difference to his parents whether he cycled or not. After a period of time his desire to impress others had morphed into a nebulous and unobtainable standard.*

*Like a black cloud looming overhead, this ideal of how he should be, how he should perform took over and there was a complete abandonment of self-trust and true self-confidence. As we worked together, he was able to let go of this external ideal, which had been dictating what to do, how to do it, when to do it, and he developed a connection and communication with his true self by directing his awareness inwards, rather than outwards.*

The development of self-trust comes as we slide along the continuum from being externally referenced to being much more internally referenced. Allowing our feelings to flow without resistance or comparison and aligning our actions with the nudges from our true self. This often goes hand in hand with moving from low consciousness to high consciousness.

# CHAPTER 5

# Who Am I Anyway?

J ANE OPENED HER EYES AND PEELED BACK THE DUVET. EVERY
bone and joint seemed to ache and creek. The light streamed in
from behind the curtains sending a searing pain from to the front of
her head to the back. She considered the effort it was going to take
just to get herself off the mattress. She braced herself and forced her
aching body upwards, taking in a sharp breath as she straightened her
back. She swung her legs off the bed and maneuvered herself around.
Even her feet hurt as they hit the floor next to the bed, how could that
be, how was it even possible that the bottoms of her feet would hurt?
With what seemed like an audible groan, she heaved herself up and
walked towards the bathroom.

As she looked in the mirror she recognized the same face that
stared back at her every day. But today was different, today she
wondered:

*"Who am I?*
*What am I?*
*What am I doing here?*
*Am I more than this?"*

There was a part of her that felt that the face looking back at her
wasn't really her, almost as if it was just a mask, hiding the real her;
whoever or whatever that was. She had a yearning to know who she
really was, to feel who she really was, to let herself flow and be free,
but she didn't know how, she didn't even know where to start.

Over the last few years, Jane had felt different. Yes, she knew that
the symptoms that flared and receded had played their part, but there
seemed to be more to it than that. There were times when life seemed

bizarre, incomprehensible, almost as if she as looking at the world through a different set of eyes. Why was life so difficult, so complicated, why couldn't it be easy, straightforward and simple. Why weren't there simple answers to her health challenges and desire for peace of mind?

Jane wanted to know who she was, beyond the superficial. She was convinced that a deeper understanding of herself would pave the way to the health and vitality that she so craved. She was concerned that she felt different from other people; she felt as if there was something stirring deep inside her, an awakening that was affecting every part of her life. Yet everyone else seemed so contented, happy to be getting on with their lives, their jobs their relationships. Was she really that different, didn't they have the same questions as her? Were they really as happy and confident as they appeared on the surface or was there more going on below that was so cleverly camouflaged from view? Weren't people worried, concerned, or even curious about what seemed like an avalanche of crises unleashing itself on the planet?

Jane wanted answers. She wanted to know how to get well, she wanted to know who she was and where she fit in. She wanted to know why she felt different, changeable, and she wanted to know, what the hell was going on.

## What On Earth Is Going On?

Are you noticing that life all around seems to be shifting at an incredibly fast pace? Does it feel like time is speeding up as you have more to do and less time to do it in? Are you experiencing changes within your own life that are either somewhat surprising or uncomfortable, or maybe you simply feel different and you can't seem to explain why?

We are currently witnessing enormous changes in every aspect of our lives and in the world around us. Much of what we are seeing appears to be turbulent, from economic chaos and financial meltdown, to bizarre anomalies within our weather systems; corruption within governments, breakdowns within societies, cultures, relationships and family systems, and overwhelm, hopelessness and confusion. On an individual level, many are experiencing confusion as their sense of identity begins to shift. This manifests itself through new and different feelings about work, relationships, and hobbies. When your identity is challenged in this way it can feel very uncomfortable and unsettling. Having the feeling that you don't enjoy your job anymore, or that your once loved hobby now just leaves you feeling empty and bored can throw you off. This is when you really begin to see how your mind has defined you and the impact that has on the way you view life. If the weekend meant coffee with particular friends or a couple of rounds of golf, and the very notion of these now leaves you a little cold, planning becomes tricky and fear can set in. Your existing identity is being challenged as it begins to expand. Of course, the first question you are likely to ask is, what is that happening to me, what on earth is going on?

In the absence of knowledge and information pertaining to the cause of these changes, a great deal of fear, drama and resentment can arise as people desperately seek stability, certainty and "normality." There can be a strong tendency to resist the discomfort and attribute it to our own failings and shortcomings. The tendency to fixate and focus upon external events can leave you feeling off-kilter and uncertain. Redirecting your focus inwards and allowing whatever takes place in life to simply unfold is less emotionally turbulent. This does not mean sticking your head in the sand, it means learning to trust your true self and begin the practice of being guided by your internal feelings towards making a positive outcome for yourself in your life. There will always be factors that lie outside of our control that will impact us, but we can remain aligned by allowing our feelings to flow rather than getting caught up in our thinking brain trying to analyze how we feel and how we can change how we feel.

In the early 20th century Russian scientist, A. L. Tchijevsky created an index of mass human excitability to understand the connection between sunspot activity and significant human activity, such as wars, revolutions, civil unrest, financial or economic crises, and the like. He found that 80 percent of significant events took place during times of maximum sunspot activity. He speculated that the sun's activity could impact upon the electrical system of the brain, affecting emotional balance and brain wave patterns among other things.

As we go through what seems like an enormous change the transition period can seem chaotic as the old systems and paradigms break down to make way for the new. The Nobel Prize–winning chemist, Ilya Prigogine, postulated that when an energy overload is introduced into a system, the system will either break down and cease to exist or it will reorganize itself to a higher level of functioning—evolve—in order to cope with the energetic input. As the system evolves to this higher level of functioning chaos can be experienced as the old breaks down and the new follows. If we look at a very simplistic real life example; if you have decided your house is too small and living arrangements are becoming uncomfortable, you might choose to add an extension to your property. When builders and contractors come in and begin work, chaos takes over during the transformational period. When the extension is complete the house is bigger and better equipped to serve the needs of your family. The same can be said for individuals; if you've ever been through a period of change at any age you'll remember that the transition state was somewhat uncomfortable. While you're going through the change it can seem like a whirlwind has carried you off, and the discomfort is never ending. If we apply this idea to the transitional period the Earth is going through, could we suggest that as we move closer towards the center of the solar system the energy overload that comes onto the planet forces a reorganization and evolution to a higher level of functioning?

As we shift from one form to another, the tendency is to go into a state of fear and worry. However, we can get trapped in fear and worry and these can compound any discomfort and slow our progress as we move through this transition. The key is to accept change; in fact, I'd go so far as to say embrace change, with curiosity and positivity, especially now.

We would all like to seek greater harmony on our planet, and, as individuals, we are a microcosm or hologram of the entire universe, so in order to see change in our world we need to start by making changes within ourselves. Despite seeming somewhat farfetched, when we change ourselves we help change the planet. Changes on a global scale have to start with changes within the individual. As more people align their body, mind, and soul, the collective effect on the energy grid of the planet has the potential to be enormous.

So you may be thinking, "Well, that's all well and nice, but what does that have to do with the pain and fatigue symptoms that I am experiencing?" As human beings, we are affected by both external and internal factors. Understanding the bigger picture and how it relates to your health and vitality is important as you being to move forward and make the changes required to achieve the life you desire.

## The Structure of Identity

Let's turn our attention to the internal factors that are affecting our sense of self. This is where we really begin to step into our empowerment space and take ownership of who we are becoming. Do you ever wonder who you really are, why you are here or where you come from? Is there a purpose to your life; is there a purpose to anyone's life? Are you your body, your brain, your personality, your soul? Or do you define yourself by your job, your achievements or your behaviors? Or maybe you feel that other people, your family, friends, teachers, work colleagues, and peers; their views, perceptions, and expectations of you define you?

If you were to stop and think about it for a moment, my guess would be that you like to think you know who you are. If I asked you to get a paper and pen and write down some words to describe or define you, what would you write? Might you list look something like this?

| | |
|---:|:---|
| Loving | Resourceful |
| Warm | Strategic |
| Friendly | Detail focused |
| Patient | A good friend |
| Helpful | An animal lover |

Or maybe your list would be more specific or more negative and critical? Whatever you write, it is going to be the result of how you see yourself. But is this notion of self, this idea of who you are that you hold in your mind actually right? And is that idea fixed or flowing?

The important notion for us to consider is the role that our sense of identity plays in our health, well-being, and our life experience. Regardless of how our identity is formed, how true it is or whether it remains fixed or is fluid, one thing is for sure and that is that our sense of identity is an extremely strong motivating force behind our behavior. Our tendency is to act in alignment with our identity even when we are not aware this is what we are doing. Depending on our level of self-awareness, our identity can be something of an iceberg in that there are aspects that we are aware of and familiar with, and aspects that we are not.

Without doubt, you will have known people who have engaged in an activity or perhaps gone traveling in order to "find themselves."

What do they mean? Well, by immersing themselves in different cultures and experiences they have the opportunity to observe themselves and feel different things, to experience themselves in different ways and therefore learn about themselves. Or you've heard famous celebrities or sports personalities talk about how they learned a great deal about themselves when faced with difficult or problematic life situations. In all these instances a little bit more of the iceberg reveals itself. A broader sense of identity is experienced and created. Because identity can be such a strong driving force and has the potential to be fluid and continually changing, developing a greater awareness brings with it an opportunity to develop it further.

The idea of learning about yourself, observing yourself and experiencing yourself is interesting when you think about it. Who is doing that observing, who is doing the feeling, who is doing the experiencing? As we discussed earlier, we have an internal drive to move away from pain or discomfort and move towards comfort or pleasure. We could suggest that everything we are doing is at some level serving us by taking us away from discomfort to comfort. As you look at everything you do in your life, whether you think it's good or bad is, at some level serving you, even when your conscious mind knows that what you are doing may not be in your best interest, the drives to maintain a sense of identity and away from discomfort to comfort are powerful. Let's use the example of smoking. Tom and Jim are buddies and they have both smoked for about 15 years. For the last five they've talked about quitting but now the time has finally come when they are going to take the plunge. They have heard others talk about the benefits not only financially, but also for mental clarity, health and overall sense of vitality, energy, and well-being. They set a start date for when they intend to quit and hope for the best. Three months later Jim has successfully quit, in fact it took little effort, far less than he was expecting, he just decided to quit and that was that. Tom, on the other hand, is still struggling, still smoking despite having tried all available options from nicotine patches to gum.

What's the difference, how is Jim able to stop and Tom not? When we look at the three areas of identity, our tendency to move towards comfort and away from discomfort, and the idea that everything we do is serving us at some level whether we are aware of it or not, an interesting picture begins to reveal itself. Tom sees himself as a smoker, it's who he is, it is part of how he defines himself. Smok-

ing is attached to his sense of identity. As we saw above, our mind
wants to hold on to a sense of identity and doesn't want this to shift.
When this sense of identity remains hidden under the surface it can
be difficult to shift. Even though Tom says he doesn't want to smoke
anymore the fact that smoking is somehow attached to his identity
makes it extremely difficult for him to quite. Jim, on the other hand,
saw smoking as a simply something he did, he never really saw himself as a smoker, it was just a behavior. Shifting a behavior is much
easier than shifting one's identity. This is not to say that identity can't
be shifted. Our identity is fluid and "we" are merely the observers;
however, manipulating it is far easier when our level of awareness is
higher.

The second point is our tendency to move towards pleasure or
comfort and away from pain and discomfort. When we have a "strategy" for alleviating "stress" or discomfort we will stick with it until
it is effectively replaced. This combines with the idea that whatever
we do is serving us at some level. For Tom, smoking was a way to
alleviate discomfort, the "stresses" and "strains" of daily life. When
Tom tried to quit he didn't replace smoking and didn't find alternative
methods to alleviate his own internal discomfort. This made giving
up extremely difficult for him. Smoking was an effective strategy for
dealing with internal discomfort by providing some internal comfort, even though Tom said he wanted to quit and was concerned
about the impact smoking was having on his health. As we discussed
in our last chapter, our emotions and feelings are the biggest drivers
for our behavior, even when we think that we are making conscious
rational choices and decisions, emotions are the secret underground
driving force.

In contrast to Tom, Jim smoked for pleasure, he was far better at
regulating and processing his own emotion so smoking did not serve
the purpose of alleviating discomfort. Jim didn't lose anything by not
smoking. He still hung out with his friends who smoked and still
engaged in all the activities that he enjoyed.

What we are beginning to see is that even though maintaining
a sense of identity protects us as we move through our day-to-day
lives, it can also inhibit us. That same sense of identity proves to be
an extremely strong driver or motivating force behind our behavior. What this means is that the unconscious sense of identity that is
securely locked inside will drive your behavior, and you will have a

tendency to align with that sense of identity even if you know that what you are doing may not be useful for you. The more you develop open awareness and connect the more obvious these drives become and the easier they are to shift when not useful.

## Daily Life: Role and Identity

When you get up in the morning, how do you know what to do? If you suffer from a fatigue, pain or other health challenges, there is a good chance you awake with symptoms, and you might believe that these dictate what you do. You probably feel that you have little or no choice because symptoms are taking over your life.

If you don't wake with symptoms, aches, pains, anxiety or depression, then how do you know what to do in the morning. If you get in the shower, what do you wash first? My guess would be that you wash in the same order every day, and some days you may not even remember what you have and haven't washed. We've all had that experience of having washed our hair yet we can't remember if we've washed our hair. Why is that? Are you going crazy if that happens?

When you get out of the shower and get dressed, you stroll over to your wardrobe, open it up and look inside. How do you know what to wear? Do you feel it, think it or just act out of impulse, almost as if you are in a trance state and you are going through the motions of daily life? When this happens how do you know who you are? Are you choosing who you are?

When I worked as a psychologist in management consulting, I would get up at the same time every day, take a shower, wash in exactly the same order, get dressed in basically the same few items that were appropriate attire for the professional world of consulting, then I'd head downstairs, eat the same breakfast, leave the house the same time and sit in traffic on the commute to work. I thought I hated work, but when I left the company to move into full-time therapy and coaching work, I realized that I didn't hate working for that company after all, in fact I really quite enjoyed it. What I actually hated was the boredom that ensued from the mindless trance state that had become my morning routine. My true self got lost as I allowed myself to float in this semi-conscious state.

Now this is a very interesting area; we know that making decisions requires a great deal of energy, and as our brains are the biggest calorie guzzlers in our body, making endless decisions can fatigue us (more about this in Chapter 11). So if I had to get up and make twenty decisions before hitting the office, there's a good chance I'd be completely exhausted by the time I got to my desk. However, by totally tuning-out I had become passive in relation to what I was doing, the result was an inertia driven boredom. Boredom plays a far greater role in most people's experience than we care to admit. There is a false notion that boredom levels relate to the amount of activity that you are doing; thus the often heard statement, "I'm too busy to be bored." However, it's entirely possible to be incredibly busy and completely bored. When this happens we either seek out experiences that will give us some sort of emotional experience, be it pleasant or unpleasant, or we tune-out and move through life in a trancelike rut.

Soldiers returning from war zones and combat often crave a return to that environment. They will also talk about the depth of the connections and friendships they make as being far stronger than anything experienced in civilian life. On the surface this may seem crazy, however, as we look a little deeper it begins to make sense. When we go through life-and-death situations an enormous amount of emotion is triggered. When we feel huge amounts of emotion we tend to bond with people who are in the same situation. As we radiate emotion through our biofield it connects with the biofields of others and bonds are formed. The stronger the emotion the stronger the bonds. If you were to stop for a moment and think about the people you feel particularly close with there is a good chance you have experienced significant emotional events together. This is one explanation as to why we retain friendships from childhood, because those early years are emotionally significant. As we get older life can get boring. This is certainly what soldiers experience when they back from war. Going from a situation where significant responsibility has to be taken for other people's lives as well extremely expensive equipment, to one where nothing really happens and there could be responsibility for almost nothing results in massive boredom and a shutting down of self. In my view this is a significant contributor to on-gong PTSD. When soldiers come home and have a sense of purpose, meaning and feel useful in their chosen pursuit, they have a rewarding emotional experience and their natural self-correcting mechanism can work. This can facilitate the reduction of PTSD symptoms naturally. However, when they are not able to find a sense of purpose, meaning and fulfillment a massive surge of boredom takes over and health is impacted as a disconnection from true self occurs. Boredom gives time to focus on symptoms and attempts to fix those symptoms often leads illness lifestyle and the ensuing spiral. I'm not pointing the finger solely at boredom, and I am not suggesting a simple solution for PTSD. I am merely making the point that the opposite of boredom is a lack of fulfillment and a sense of fulfillment is what arises the more we align with our true self.

The point of this is to raise your awareness about the need for experience in life, the need to be active players in our lives, making choices that are right for us. Automating certain decisions can be valuable, but not at the expense of awareness. If we completely tune-out there is every chance that our identity is dictated by our conditioning, our environment, and other people, we become bored and this has a significant impact on health and symptoms levels. I would invite you to take a look at and change your daily routine, freshen it up and align it more with something that allows you to feel alive. Feeling alive means you are aligning with your true self.

## Illness and Identity

One of the significant implications of living with a major health challenge is the impact it has on your sense of identity. If you have experienced symptoms of pain or fatigue, anxiety or depression and feel powerless to change or alleviate them, there can be a ripple effect impacting all aspects of your perception of yourself and your abilities. Identity is a complex issue that develops and evolves over time as our natural "wiring" interacts with the world around us. Often our ideas about who we are can differ from the deeper truth about who we are. When we get knocked off course and deviate from our true self, we end up being more of who we are not as our mind reviews who we've been and projects that out into the future. When we experience something for a prolonged period of time this has the potential to significantly impact our identity without us realizing. If you have suffered from a health challenge for a long time and you have built your life around having symptoms there is a very strong chance that your behavior will have started to morph into your identity.

What are the signs that you may have developed an illness identity? If you stop for a moment and review your life and the activities in your life, how many of those things would you still do if you were perfectly healthy and there were no signs of the problems you currently experience? How many friends and acquaintances do you have who also have the same or similar health challenges? Do you notice yourself saying, "my chronic fatigue," or "my fibromyalgia," or "my anxiety and depression," or "my IBS"? If you do, then there is a good chance that your symptoms have become part of your sense of identity. If this continues to be the case, shifting those symptoms might prove harder than if they are not part of your identity. Of course, this begs the question of, how do I shift them?

Whatever symptoms you experience, they are not you, they are an experience, a process, they are feedback, they are not *you*. You are so much more, more than you can currently envisage or even comprehend. You are far more than your current conception of yourself. You are more than you see in the mirror and you are more than your behaviors, actions, words, thoughts, feelings, and reactions.

## The Metaphysical Perspective

Do you feel that you are more than your physical body? Do have a sense that there is something greater than you that exists outside or beyond you? Do you think you have a soul? What do you think happens when you cease to exist in human form? From quantum theorists to spiritual sages, there is a prevailing theme that we are more than merely flesh and bone. Rather we are vibrational beings and the level of our vibration and the frequencies we radiate impact not only the world around us but also the nature of reality itself.

When I became interested in metaphysical and spiritual ideas and concepts, an idea that seemed to crop up over and over again was that it can be very hard "trying" to be spiritual when you're a human being. Spirituality seemed to be something you strived for and achieved as long as you put certain practices into action and dedicated yourself to implementing habits, while at the same time eliminating others. There was an idea that being spiritual meant sacrificing and suffering in order to reach a goal of enlightened bliss, transcending being human. None of this made any sense to me and felt somewhat strange; why would we have to suffer and sacrifice?

I then came across the idea that we are spiritual beings having the experience of being human. This really resonated with me; it made

complete sense that rather than thinking of ourselves as human trying to be spiritual, we are spiritual beings playing at being human. It's
not about escaping being human and trying to be spiritual, we already
are spirit. So, we could suggest that the true path to being spiritual is
to fully engage with life, embrace the true essence of being human,
and live the full expression of who you really are. The more we can
align with our true self the more freedom we experience and the less
we are constricted by health challenges.

Every experience you have is important, your past experiences
not only energetically and vibrationally reside within your unconscious mind and energy fields, they also reside within the collective
energy fields—you leave an energetic imprint wherever you go. As
you begin to shift your vibration and take charge of your life, you are
impacting upon the vibration and energy of the entire planet. Sounds
exciting, doesn't it.

# CHAPTER 6

# The Expanded Self

## The Thinker and the Feeler

HOW MUCH TIME DO YOU SPEND THINKING ABOUT THE past, going over situations and conversations? How much time do you spend thinking about the future, "what if-ing" about events or circumstances: "What if this happens?" or "What if that doesn't happen?" "What if she says this, or if he says that?" "What if I can't cope? What if I can't do it? What if I get it wrong? What if they don't like me? What if I'm not good enough?" Does that sound familiar?

As a culture, our primary focus is on thinking. Thinking is viewed as the pinnacle of human endeavor, the solver of problems, the pathway out of suffering. As a result, we have a tendency to focus our energy and attention in our head, to think about everything; to analyze, scrutinize, seek meaning in emotions and situations, and base decisions on what we think, without balancing that with what we feel or know deep down. The irony is that as we have seen, emotion affects all our thinking, so even when we think we are making an emotion-free decision, it is still influenced by emotion at some level.

Our schooling systems predominantly focus on developing analytical thinking skills, commonly referred to as "left-brain" skills. The conveyer belt of mainstream education churns out young people whose emotional and spiritual intelligence is left largely untouched and undeveloped. Interestingly, as children go through kindergarten into primary (preschool), and beyond their ability for divergent thinking diminishes dramatically. Divergent thinking is the method used to generate creative ideas in order to identify or generate many possible solutions. Divergent thinking is nonlinear, creative, free-flowing. Its opposite, convergent thinking, is about following a correct sequence in order to find one correct answer. Divergent thinking is something of a "whole-brain" activity in that it requires both left and right hemispheres, compared with convergent thinking, which is far more "left-brain" oriented. I put inverted commas around whole-brain and left-brain because there is still debate within the world of neuroscience as to exactly what areas of the brain are used in different types of thinking.

Whole brain pursuits activate insight, intuition and inner-knowing. These are part and parcel of our identity; however, as children grow our education system fails to foster and develop these natural tendencies, and trains children to focus their energy and attention on their memory development and analytical thinking faculties to the detriment of intuition and insight. We know that who we are, our sense of self and identity comprises all these aspects of ourselves, so the neglect of intuition, emotion, and inner wisdom inhibits our ability to experience ourselves. Our identity has the capacity to continually develop and evolve through our lifetime. There is no single "me," rather a series of potentials that are impacted by my natural "wiring," experience, focus and environment. It is a trap to think that what we think or what we feel *is* who we are, or that we remain exactly the same throughout our lifetime. What you think and what you feel form part of your experience but neither are the totality of you. Your true self is expansive and all encompassing. You can observe what you feel and observe what you think without drowning in either or allowing either to dominate your sense of self. Feelings are feedback and thoughts are just experience.

## The Brain as a Tool

Attaching our identity to our thoughts is one of our biggest errors we make that leads us down a path of battling thoughts and feeling emotionally uncomfortable or symptomatic. We don't consciously do this, in fact, for the most part, we are not aware that this is what we are doing, which is why need to consciously go through a process of realizing that we are assuming we are our thoughts and they are absolutely true. Thoughts lead to a version of reality that we are choosing to create at a single point in time. They are not representative of some "absolute reality," some concrete fixed notion of what is.

There is no absolute objective reality; there are merely points of perception and meanings that we attribute to those points of perception. Confusion usually arises because the "facts" or markers of reality we agree upon vary. Objectivity and subjectivity have been staples of philosophy since the origins of rational thought, so I am not seeking to take a deep journey into the philosophical underpinning of life, rather I'm inviting you to adopt a simplistic existentialist view. The perspective that it is humans who define the meaning in life and not life defining its own meaning.

For our purposes separating our thoughts for our total sense of identity is important. Rational thinking is a skill and a useful technique, but recognizing that it is not the totality of us is an important distinction. Here's an idea, could you allow yourself to think of your thinking brain as a tool you use, a bit like your computer, rather than all of who you are? When the time is right to analyze, apply critical reasoning and logic you can recruit your thinking brain. It's a little bit like using the right piece of cutlery for the right dish. My guess is that you don't eat soup with a fork; so you shouldn't try to use the thinking brain to analyze your intuitive and emotional experience, or try to figure out who you are.

The same can be true of feelings; it can be easy to attach your identity to your feelings and assume they mean something about you and who you are; or even that you *are* those feelings. These could be feelings in your body, such as tension, or sensations in your mind like misty bleakness. While they form part of you they are not the totality of you, they are an experience you are having. You are not the experience you are having, you are observing the experience. They do not mean anything about you; they are simply feedback. When we have negative feelings in life there can be a tendency to either resist those feelings or feel that you will drown in them. This could be anything from feeling inadequate, to feeling fearful, sad or unhappy. You are not what you feel, but at the same time it is vital that you are in your body to pay attention to what you feel so that you may be guided where necessary.

Let's do a quick experiment: Think of a recent memory that you can fully re-associate with, i.e. see what you could see at the time, hear what you could hear, and feel what you could feel. This could be any memory, but I would suggest a pleasant one; maybe a trip to the beach or a park, something pleasant. Allow yourself to become immersed in the memory and while you see, hear and feel everything that is going on in that memory, allow yourself to simply observe what you see, hear and feel. Imagine expanding so you encompass all you see, hear and feel, while observing and not attaching yourself it any of it, almost as if you are looking in, having the experience while observing the experience, aware that it is taking place. Maybe you could imagine floating slightly backwards and upwards where you can still fully experience everything coming into your senses, while opening up to the idea that this sensory "data" is not the totality of you. This is where you can begin to practice open awareness, observing, feeling, sensing but not getting pulled in.

This observation comes from the expanded you, which is aligned with your true self. This expanded space is greater than your physical body and extends into your biofield. Imagine that the expanded you is able to notice everything and experience everything that takes place within your physical body and brain at the same time. Let yourself expand into this space and notice what it feels like to know that you are much bigger, much more expansive than you currently think.

Don't try to define yourself in this expanded space, simply practice entering this space with open awareness as you observe your thoughts and feelings, fully experiencing everything in your life, knowing that you are more than you think, more than you see and more than you feel. When you move into this expanded space that is within and beyond your physical body, you can acknowledge and experience everything that takes place without judgment, without resistance. This is crucially important because the judgment and resistance cause significant blockages of energy and flow.

## How to Experience the Expanded Self

Have you ever played a game and become so absorbed in that game that you completely lost yourself, almost like your body was taken over by the emotion of the game? The intensity is so great it's almost suffocating; you are completely focused, and completely engrossed in the drama of the game as it unfolds before your eyes. Then you have a realization that it is only a game. As you have this realization, somehow, an expanded perspective reveals itself where you see the game for what it is, just a game. This doesn't

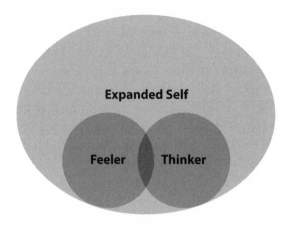

diminish your felt-sense experience, the emotions you feel, or the enjoyment you are deriving from playing the game. This experience propels you into a different perspective, almost as if you go from being immersed to being able to experience and observe, like you are looking down when floating on a cloud, while at the same time being completely connected to all the feelings and sensations in your body. You shift into a perception that is different; it's more expansive and flexible, it's less cramped and stifling. You can still feel all the emotion, while knowing you are not controlled by it—it is, after all, only a game.

What if you were able to do this with life? What if you knew deep down in your true self that life was merely a game that you were playing? Even though life can seem so real and so serious it is just a game where you are playing at having the experience of yourself. Every emotion you feel is simply feedback, not something to be analyzed through mental rumination, merely something to guide your actions where appropriate.

You might think it's a strange notion, but what if you somehow knew that life what just a game and nothing actually mattered? What do you think you would feel? If you can allow yourself to play with that feeling for a moment, you'll probably experience resistance to it. Most people have difficulty entertaining the idea that nothing really matters, and of course when it comes to actual life we have imprinted meaning on so many things that there will be people, places and circumstances that do seem to matter. However, you might find that your emotional experience begins to change when you open into and embrace your expanded self. Allowing yourself to feel without resistance, while spending a little more time with open awareness in the present and a little less time in your head jumping between the past and the future can have a significant impact on your life experience. You won't be so concerned when circumstances deviate or don't turn out as you had planned. You'll flow with it rather than pushing against it, and this will seem a little bit like things don't matter as much. This flexibility is you in your Energy-flow, allowing life to happen, experiencing it as it happens knowing that everything that happens is okay. We will talk more about removing judgment and the implications of that in Chapter 8. For now, allow yourself to play with and enjoy the idea of your expanded self.

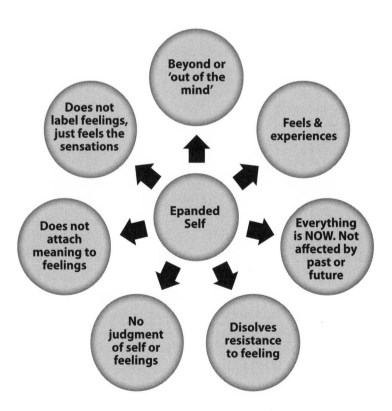

## An Unfolding Reality

If you were to stop and think about it for a moment, my guess is that you would probably agree that there is some sort of objective reality "out there," and that what takes place in your head could be seen to be an accurate representation of that reality. What if you were to entertain the idea that there are an almost infinite number of potential realities all coexisting? The reality that you experience is unfolding now and arises from your point of perception. You are quite literally co-creating your experience of reality on a moment-by-moment basis. As your perception changes so does your experience of reality.

We often assume that everything that happens in our head is a true reflection of a single reality that exists out there in life. If the little voice in your head tells you that you have wasted ten years in a job, that you are useless and your life is pretty worthless, you believe it because you think that little voice is *you*, you think it is reality. Rather than recognizing that this is a point of perception that impacts your experience of reality and affects your decision-making and ongoing behavior. If you remember earlier in the book we talked about how what exists outside us and what exists inside us, in our body and brain, are a flowing interconnected system, not two separate mutually exclusive entities. We are influencing our environment and our environment is influencing us. The more you can allow yourself to embrace this notion the less trapped you will feel in life, the more expansive and free you will feel. Your life is an unfolding reality on a moment by moment basis and you are driving the bus.

I know that for many years I didn't even question whether the little voice in my head was me. I assumed there as a single reality and that life was happening to me. The more educated I was the more I became locked in my head, the more I analyzed absolutely everything about life. Between ages seventeen and twenty-four I went from being a partial resident to a full-time resident in my thinking brain. I analyzed my own analysis and as a result I was completely dysfunctional. I experienced high levels of anxiety and depression and spent my time analyzing why. I didn't realize that this was something I was doing, a process I was going through. It didn't occur to me that I had the ability to change this experience. I assumed that I was the thinker who was doing the thinking and that the output of this thinking was a reflection of a single objective reality. I continued to apply the same method of attempting to solve my problems—thinking—without knowing that this attempted solution was exacerbating and amplifying the anxiety I was experiencing. I unconsciously assumed that my perceptions of the "out there" reality were also true. The notion that my reality was a result of my chosen point of perception would have probably sent me reeling.

Our identity is often very closely aligned with what is taking place in our thinking brain or mind and the way that connects with our notion of a single objective reality. I often hear people say things like, "Yeah, but that's not reality, is it," especially when referring to a celebrity or entertainer; or on returning home after a vacation its, "Well, I'm back to reality." The point is that the reality is defined by the experiencer, it is not something that is objective requiring a consensus of agreement. Your reality is your reality, created largely by you, because outside and inside are not separate, they are interwoven and connected. The "facts" of your life take their meaning from the feelings you attach to them and thus reality is born. We believe we are the thinker and that what the thinker says is true. When this thinking becomes erratic and seemingly out of control, conventional methods seek to tame the beast of thought, to subtly alter from negative to positive.

But what is needed is something more profound so we can begin to understand who we are in relation to the thinking that has the potential to run riot and take over our lives completely. You are not your thinking brain, and the output of your thinking brain is not simply a reflection of a single reality. Even though we cannot dominate and control our thinking, we know that it is hugely influenced and colored by our emotion.

What if you were to allow yourself to recognize three crucially important pieces of information:

1. The thinking that takes place in your head is affected by your current emotion, your recent thinking habits and "thought energy" or "mass consciousness" (more about this shortly), that it is not a representation of absolute truth, and not you.
2. There is no single objective reality, your experience of reality unfolds in front of you on a moment-by-moment basis and is significantly influenced by your point of perception.

3. What we are going to call "you" is more than just your thinking brain. You are a cascading series of interwoven and overlapping energies intermingling with the energy of everything around you—the expanded self, your true self.

The picture below is a representation of the energy bodies or energy fields that form part of who we are, our expanded self. The arrows represent the flow of influence, with each energy-body impacting the energy-bodies below. There is some flow of influence up the pyramid but it is not as significant as the flow down the pyramid. An example of this being that creative visualization can increase muscle strength—the mental energy-body impacting the physical energy-body. There was a piece of research that looked at finger strength and found that visualization and exercise both resulted in significant differences in strength as compared to a control group. It's also been shown that a specific visualization exercise can lead to an increase in white blood cell count. Both these are examples that the mental energy-body exerts a significant influence over the physical energy-body. We learned in our chapter on emotion that there are more connections from the heart to the brain than the other way around, and we have seen that emotional processing is faster than cognitive processing, so we are concluding that the emotional energy-body has a significant influence over the mental body. There is some influence of the mental on the emotional; however, it is nothing like as significant. In practice, this means that our thinking is not going to exert a significant impact on our natural flowing emotion and we are not going to change our emotions by just changing our thoughts. This also explains why when people have profound awakenings, like near death experiences, their entire lives change.

## Thinking, Memory, and You

When we review the nature and content of thinking, a significant chunk involves reviewing the past, projecting into the future, or ruminating over scenarios that somehow always seem to reflect badly on you. The thinking that involves digging into the past involves access to memories to recall and go over events from the past. Contrary to popular belief, the brain does not act as a filing cabinet or computer where a memory is stored in tact and filed away to be retrieved when

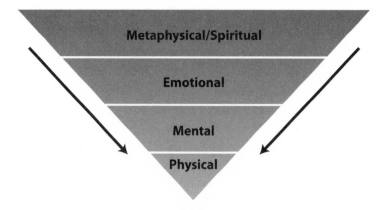

needed. As we have learned, emotion affects everything, and this includes our memory storage and retrieval.

In order to recall a memory we have to recreate the neural pathways within the brain. Memories are not simply stored, they have to be recreated each time and because the manner of our thinking is impacted by our emotional state, the nature of the recreation of the memory will be affected by the emotion we have attached to that memory. This means that the potential for memory distortion is significant. The more emotion attached to a memory the stronger the attachment to that memory and the greater the likelihood for a distortion from actual events.

The area of the brain most associated with memory is the hippocampus. This is a small organ located within the brain's medial temporal lobe and forms part of the traditional limbic system. As these areas of the brain are most likely impacted with HPA dysfunction it is no surprise that if you suffer from a chronic fatigue or pain condition, or even anxiety or depression symptoms, you may experience problems of memory formation and retrieval. Mainstream science has consistently struggled to find a single location for memory within the brain, only areas that are involved in memory formation and retrieval. Karl Spencer Lashley worked at Harvard University in 1950s and much of his research dealt with the role of the cerebral cortex in learning and memory. In what has become something of a classic series of experiments, Lashley sought to identify the specific areas of the brain involved in learning in rats. The experiments involved training rats to run a maze then remove certain areas of the cerebral cortex and see if the rat could remember the maze. Much to the amazement of the researchers, as much as 50 percent of a rat's cerebral cortex could be removed and have little impact on the rat's ability to run the maze remembering which route to take. The conclusions were that memory for a task does not reside in any single fixed location within the brain.

The biologist Rupert Sheldrake and the psychologist, Professor Gary Schwartz have suggested that the brain acts more like receiver transmitter than a storage facility and that memories exist as vibrational potentials in quantum fields outside the brain. Sheldrake has developed the Carl Jung idea of a collective unconscious and suggested that learning and memory in nature are more like habits that he calls morphic resonance, where information exists as nonmaterial potentials within morphic fields. This theory suggests that there is no memory bank that exists to deliver perfect, in tact objective memories. Like thoughts, our memories exist as vibrational potentials that we create and recreate, and the nature of their creation is dependent upon our vibration, our feeling state.

When we look at our own experience of memory it seems to make perfect sense. The more we revisit and recreate a memory the stronger the emotional charge and the more biased and distorted it becomes. The memory fields are continually recreated and each time they are modified depending on the emotional charge that drives the thinking. We think these memories are a true representation of objective reality and base decisions and life choices on these memories.

In my early days working with sufferers of CFS and fibro, I had a period where I seemed to attract a number of sufferers who experienced early life abuse. The experiences of these sufferers and the questions they posed were identical. They reported that, along with the physical symptoms of CFS and fibro, they also experienced involuntary memories that haunted them. These memories would jump into their minds out of nowhere. They were distressing and traumatic. The question being, how could we get rid of them. Having trained in a number of therapeutic modalities including hypnotherapy and the meridian tapping therapy, TFT, and having had some informal training in *eye movement desensitization and reprocessing* (EMDR), I told my clients that we would deal with their physical symptoms of CFS and fibro then following that we would come back and work on their post-traumatic memory symptoms.

When we got to the point when the physical symptoms were almost gone, this cluster of clients reported that the involuntary memories were all but gone as well. One client said, "It's weird those memories just don't haunt me anymore, in fact they never jump into my mind. If I think about it, I can consciously recreate them but even then even though they are not pleasant, they seem further away and don't have any sort of hold over me. They almost seem separate from me, detached somehow."

How could this be? We hadn't done any work on trying to process or get rid of those involuntary memories, yet these clients were telling me that even conscious re-creation of the memories did not trigger anything like the level of emotional discomfort that had been experienced. The experience connects with what we discussed in Chapter 2 about PTSD.

As I allowed myself to process this information, two flashes of insight came to me. First, that maybe memories served as a tap on the shoulder in much the same way as symptoms did. Something was happening right now, emotion was present, and probably being missed or blocked somehow. Memories connected to similar frequency emotions were then being "presented" to conscious awareness as a means of attracting attention. So maybe emotion radiates frequency in much the same way and then resonates with older memories.

Have you ever had the experience of looking through older photographs of yourself? As you browse there will be some photographs that immediately pull you back in time. It's as if it were yesterday, you completely associate with the younger you and remember everything about the situation or event. Then there are other photographs that you cannot even believe that you are looking at yourself in the picture. You have little memory of it, or what memory you do have seems grainy and way off in the distance. The reason you can't associate with that younger you in the photo and you find it hard to remember the event is because some aspects of you have shifted, your vibration is different from the person in the picture.

As we are beginning to see, what is important is the now moment and everything that occurs now is happening for us not to us. So if you do have memories that spring into your mind they are doing so for a reason, you are resonating with some version of you or some event in the past. Conventional psychology calls this "state dependent memory." This is why when you go out and buy your Christmas tree and get your decorations out of the boxes in the attic, any memories that pop into your mind are of previous Christmases. You are very unlikely to be putting candy-cane on the tree and have memories of lying on a beach in Summer appear in your mind.

## Tricks of the Mind

We've learned that memories will pop into our mind because they vibrationally resonate with an emotion attached to a previous experience or "version" of you. This is just one of the ways in which your mind can play tricks on you. Even though we have talked about the significant impact of emotion on thinking, the picture is deeply complex. Emotion, thinking, behavior and our environment are inextricably linked and this can make life confusing when trying to figure out what exactly what and how we feel.

One thing is for sure, and that's our emotion will affect the nature of our thinking. If the emotion in your emotional stress bucket is negative the flavor of your thoughts will be negative. The added interest is that the more you visit a particular thought the stronger the attraction to that thought, and the quicker your mind will go to that particular thought. That may sound a little confusing so here's an example.

> Despite having a good job, Tom, like many people, had financial concerns. He would frequently find himself worrying about money when in shower, when writing emails or cooking dinner. There wasn't anything particularly concrete about the nature or structure of Tom's thoughts, they crept up and manifest in an irregular nebulous sort of way. All he knew was that he'd get lost in them and they didn't feel good. He assumed, as most do, that the thoughts were a true and objective version of reality. What he didn't know was that each time he allowed himself to get caught up in these thoughts he was feeding them, strengthening them and increasing the likelihood that they would return.
>
> One Thursday, Tom was giving a training course at work, with a colleague. His colleague, Tony had a tendency to talk over Tom and interrupt when he was talking to the group. This, according to Tom, was perfectly okay and the training course was well received. Tom left work straight after the course, and as a sufferer of CFS, he noticed his symptoms begin to increase

*subtly. As he got in his car and started to drive he started to think about money and the usual concerns started to whirl around his head. Before too long his symptoms had dramatically increased. As he was telling me, Tom was convinced that his negative thinking caused his symptoms. I, on the other hand, suggested that his intelligent body wasn't overly happy that Tony was interrupting and the frustration and agitation that ensued got shoved down in Tom's emotional stress bucket. It was this suppressed emotion that initially triggered the symptoms and crucially it also triggered thinking. Because the emotion was low vibrational—agitation and frustration—it triggered negative thoughts. Tom's most frequently visited thought-form was about money, so this was the first thought that popped back into his head. As he internally pontificated about his financial woes his emotional stress bucket got fuller and symptoms increased.*

The lesson we're learning here is that when a thought pops into your head that is not directly relevant to what is taking place right now, there is a good chance that it is one of your most frequently revisited thoughts. We all have certain thoughts that seem to pop up with monotonous regularity that often relate to self-image, self-doubt, financial worries, career or job concerns. While these thoughts may represent unresolved issues that are sitting at the bottom of your stress bucket, in many instances they remain unresolved because the drone of thinking is like a mind-loop that plays over and over and is rarely related to what is taking place right now. You could be sat on a train getting bored and that boredom triggers your thoughts about self-doubt because those are the thoughts that you have been entertaining and therefore strengthening all week. They can take hold of your consciousness and conception of reality and impact your current mood pushing you down the consciousness spectrum and affecting your ongoing behavior.

What's the solution? The first step is to recognize that thinking in many instances might be triggered or exacerbated by the presence of emotion, and that emotion is feedback about the nature of your interaction with your environment right now. The second is to gently encourage your attention back to now through open awareness and feeling into the expanded self. Look at what you are doing and what your intelligent body is trying to give you a nudge about. If you can see what is going on under your nose you might be able to take some action to act on the emotion and change something about what you are doing.

## The Limitations of Changing Thought Patterns

When I started out in therapy I adopted a predominantly cognitive approach to my therapeutic interventions, and so my initial work was based on changing thinking patterns and cognitive schema, i.e., what goes on inside your head. I would spend hours getting my clients to change their internal pictures, change the nature and structure of their internal chatter and dialogue and play with other internal habits that make up thinking. I watched as clients struggled to manipulate and maneuver images and sounds in their minds. However, what became apparent was that it took an enormous amount of effort to change thinking patterns, and this effort had to be continually applied. What's more, the resulting impact on a person's life and symptoms felt unsatisfactory to me, and to my clients. On some occasions there was a positive outcome from this mental manipulation, but often there wasn't. I always tried everything on myself first, be that something I was developing myself or a technique, tool or process that I had been taught or read about. It seemed vitally important to me that if I was going to be congruent in teaching a method to a client I had to be satisfied with the efficacy of that method. When it came to working on the internal workings of my own head I just couldn't really do it. I had never been good at visualization. I was aware that my brain could create fantastic visual images but never through force or willpower. Whenever I had attended an event and been invited to go through a creative visualization exercise, I always felt a degree of frustration as I worked hard at getting the right image. Yet I knew that there were times when images would be in my mind with great clarity and precision.

Surely I couldn't be the only person who struggled to visualize at will, I'm just not that special. My sense was that if concentrated visualization and other mental manipulation techniques were not only difficult but also downright frustrating for me, they would be for others like me. So I abandoned those techniques. I'm not saying these techniques don't work, I'm merely suggesting that they are of limited utility to a percentage of the population.

Looking back it seems obvious, you can't move beyond thinking by thinking; and thinking is not the answer to everything, in fact in many instances it simply makes things worse. I was listening to a podcast recently and the host was talking about moving towards authenticity and authentic living. This sounded okay and on the right track, until she started telling people to sit down and think about who they were. "No," I thought. I wanted to get on air right there and tell her listeners not to sit down and "think" about who they were. This is exactly the problem, we have this deep-seated belief that thinking is the path to everything from solving science problems to enlightenment. Wisdom comes from figuring out where to appropriately apply your thinking skills. I can categorically tell you that you will not attain wisdom or enlightenment through thinking, and you will not experience the fullness of all you are through thinking. So please, if, like me you do love to listen to podcasts, please don't sit and think about who you are, let who you are emerge and trust your true self to flow freely.

In saying all that, it is important that we understand both the role of thinking what triggers it, so . . .

## What Triggers Thinking?

As I continued my research and practice, I began to see that dysfunctional or negative thinking patterns had a cause. The common belief seems to be that no one really knows what triggers or causes thinking, it just happens, I'm not entirely in agreement with this, in the same way as I'm not in agreement with the idea that you can simply change your thinking by getting in your head and performing some sort of mental manipulation tactics.

There are three primary triggers or causes of thinking.

1. THE PRESENCE OF EMOTION. When emotion is present in our body-mind system the cogs of the thinking brain will churn into action. This can be obvious—for example when we are driving and someone cuts into our lane, we feel a flash of anger in our body and the thinking brain goes into overdrive. It can start with a simple thought like, "what is he doing driving like that," and before long the thinking is beginning to spread. It's almost like lighting a fuse that could start with you lambasting the other driver with your internal dialogue and

end up with you ruminating over all the mistakes you have made in your life leading to this point. If you have a tendency to be remotely self-critical, and many people I have worked with (including myself) can associate with this trait; then you will know how easy it is to move from thinking about something small to wondering how did you manage to mess up that job interview, or become such a loser, or is any of it really worth it. The point I am making is that negative emotion will trigger thinking and there's a good chance that you might not feel the emotion before the thinking kicks in. In fact, you could be having some negative thoughts at any point and not really know why they are there. Because you tend to believe your thinking is true and attach it to your identity, you'll probably get caught up in the thinking without realizing it's been triggered and colored by emotion. If your thinking is negative there is a very strong possibility that the emotion that was present before the thinking was negative as well. The only difference between the two is that the emotion will be related to your interaction with your environment right now, whereas your thinking can go all over the place, like an inflated balloon that's just been released and you stand back and watch it spin and twist at top speed.

Boredom is a great example where the emotion can creep up on you and ignite your thinking brain into a machine that spurts tirades of abuse that are generally aimed at you. I've heard so many people tell me that they are too busy to be bored. But boredom is not a measure of activity level, it's a measure of the amount of fulfillment you are deriving from your activity. So you could be doing absolutely nothing and completely fulfilled in that moment, or conversely, you could have a day jam-packed with "to-dos" that all leave your intelligent-body tapping you on the shoulder with boredom. Will you feel the boredom? You may, or you might just notice that your head begins to run riot, or you could experience an increase in your symptom level. Have you ever had that experience of finding yourself mentally criticizing friends, then family, or maybe something you heard on the news two days ago; either way your mind is swerving from one item to the next taking swipe, attacking or berating. If you get a moment of clarity you may wonder how it started. How did you end up thinking about your neighbors new fence and how it irritated you when you started thinking about needing to pump up your car tires. Chances are it all started with some boredom as you were going about your chores, but you didn't feel the boredom. The emotion gets blocked, you slip down the consciousness spectrum, which impacts your perceptions of life, the emotion triggers thinking, and you're away.

2. HABIT: THE MORE WE THINK THE MORE WE THINK. As I talked about earlier, the more we think the stronger the connection we create with a thought or memory field. You will even find that the more you think about something the greater the possibility of waking up at night with the same thought going on in your head. A few years ago a client of mine was recovering from CFS working with me and following a long period of inactivity he had started to cycle again. He had four bikes and one was broken so he was fixing it. The interesting part was that he was going to work thinking about his bike, searching for parts and looking on forums and thinking a bit more about his bike. He'd get home for dinner and as his girlfriend would chat about her day he'd be thinking about his bike. Then he found he was waking up a night thinking about his bike. After a couple of nights he twigged what was going on, so he removed his focus from his bike, brought himself back into the present moment and paid greater attention to everything that was going on here and now. Almost immediately he stopped waking up at night thinking about his bike, but also he was beginning to break the habit of thinking.

As we will investigate later in the book, the more we give something attention the more life we breathe into it, the more we feed it. Thinking is exactly like this, the more we indulge in thinking, the more time we allow ourselves to become embroiled in it, churning and ruminating, the stronger the connection and attraction and the greater the likelihood of returning to the same thoughts over and over.

Habits are pretty easy to form and the habit of thinking is one many of us are familiar with. However, breaking the habit of thinking is not like breaking other habits because we can't really control our thinking. What we are able to manage is our awareness and our attention. We are never going to stop ourselves thinking and that is not the point of the exercise here. I know there are many books and programs that advocate taking control of your thinking, but in my experience, and I'm guessing yours as well, you can't control your thinking like you could your nutritional input or what TV channel you are going to watch. Thinking is not something that lies within your control. What you can do is impact the amount of thinking that takes place to a degree by redirecting your attention and allowing yourself to be more present with whatever you are doing at a given moment in time.

3. FREE-FLOATING "THOUGHT-ENERGY." This is the most esoteric of our three triggers. There is absolutely no scientific evidence whatsoever for the idea of "free-floating-thought-energy"; however, academics Rupert Sheldrake and Gary Schwartz, among others, have suggested that the brain acts like a receiver-transmitter that detects and decodes information and then projects it. In much the same way as your television or radio set are able to tune-into certain frequencies decode the data and transmit it in audio and visual format. The television and radio programs do not exist in the TVs and radios, the job of your TV and radio is to decode and transmit.

What if your brain worked in much the same way? Sheldrake has proposed a theory of memory suggesting that memory exists in morphic fields as potentials rather than in the brain itself. The idea of existing as potentials can be a difficult one to wrap your head around. The easiest way to think about this would be to imagine you are holding two tuning forks of the same frequency. If you strike the one tuning fork and it begins to "sing" the second tuning fork will also begin to "sing," if there any other tuning forks present that were not the same note they would remain silent, their "song" existing only as a potential. The same would happen if you struck your tuning fork next to a guitar and the tuning fork was in resonance with one of the guitar strings; it would emit a sound. The sound always exists as a potential and that potential is activated through frequency.

The suggestion then is that there's no big data bank in the sky, where we go and collect our memories. As our brains "tune into" those the morphic or quantum fields, our brains decode the information and the resulting experience manifests as sensory data in our mind and body—images, sounds, then feelings.

Despite being something of a paradigm shift, the idea that memory and thoughts could exist as fields puts an entirely different perspective on the nature of our thinking. To begin with it would seem to follow that we are continually creating memory and thoughts both individually and collectively. If there are collective fields, mass consciousness if you will, it would make sense that when we tune-into these fields we are influenced by the frequencies that are detected.

This is certainly a difficult concept to grasp and raises more questions than it answers. But the notion that we could be tuning-into vibrational thought-fields that are not our own could lead to the assertion they are decoded frequencies rather than absolute truths or reality. It could be that our brains are being bombarded with frequencies, some of which are decoded and transmitted into our conscious awareness and some not.

Have you ever had the experience where thoughts pop into your head that are abstract, obscure or maybe don't seem like they belong to you? Or maybe you've had the experience where old thoughts seem to appear from nowhere and get churned around like they're in a cement mixer going round and round? If we are tuning into frequencies and "mass consciousness" then this could offer an explanation for some of the more random goings on in our heads.

The crucial difference between these thoughts and those triggered by habit and emotion is that their appearance does lie largely beyond our control. However, what lies within our control is the extent to which we take ownership of these thoughts as representations of us. When we begin to see them as slightly separate from us and part of our experience in this moment rather than "this is me, this is true," we can appreciate them as transient entities, like floating clouds in the sky. As you practice feeling into the Expanded Self, you will find it easier to "observe" thoughts without having to control them or battle them. The more you can do this the less destructive they become. The more you try to control thoughts or battle with them the stronger you make them, the more you own them and the more constricted you become.

## What Drives Thinking Onwards?

If we are to assume that there is a reason, a purpose for everything that we do and everything that takes place within us, then there must be a reason for continued thinking once it has been triggered. Over and above the three original triggers, the primary driver of thinking is that at some level we believe that we need to think in order to solve or resolve the presence of emotion, to get rid of the emotion.

Let me explain this in more detail. So far we have covered the idea that when emotion is triggered for whatever reason the activity of our thinking brain naturally increases. The argument for this would be that emotion is present to offer feedback and nudge us in a particular direction and thinking could help with that. We know that negative emotion, or emotional pain, sees the brain "light-up" in similar ways to having the experience of physical pain, and as beings who are driven to move away from discomfort towards comfort it would seem obvious that we are going to try and escape our emotional discomfort. The problem that arises is that rather than using our thinking to figure out the most effective or constructive way to act in alignment with our true self, it tends to get caught up in loops analyzing, trying to solve or find meaning in our emotion.

Whether it be going over a conversation in your head, or ruminating on something that is happening at work or in your local community, thinking can take over. What frequently happens is that we will be engaged in one activity while giving a portion of our attention to ruminating and mental churning, all the time strengthening our connection to those thought fields. Here's the key learning that we need to integrate as we understand the nature and role of thinking in relation to our emotion and health.

- When our intelligent body sends emotion that is uncomfortable we tend to resist it, try to find meaning it, analyze it, or try to solve it or resolve it—which usually results in a massive increase in thinking.
- Thinking never solves emotion, it almost always makes it worse (it takes us down towards lower consciousness).
- Emotion does not need to be solved or resolved because it is not a problem. Your emotion is never a problem; it is simply guiding you back to your true self. So when we feel emotion it is a tap on the shoulder reminding us to act from our true self in this situation. We need to feel the emotion, acknowledge it and act where necessary.
- Remember that the purpose of our actions is that we are being true to ourselves, being authentic in that moment. The action should not be to try and get rid of the emotion it should be to express your true self in that moment.
- Emotion does not need to be thought about—the more

we think the more we move away from our true self and the more our vibration drops. Constructive action does sometimes need to be thought about, but that is more about working on a strategy for what we are going to do—more about this is Part II

## Steps

1. Everything you feel is okay. All the emotions and physical sensations in your body are okay. When I first had this realization it was a game changer for me. I realized how often I was resisting my emotional feelings in subtle yet consistent ways. I could see that I just assumed that negative emotion meant there as a problem and my body would tense. Just reminding myself that it was okay for me to feel, I could let myself feel the sensations, was huge.

2. Your emotion is never a problem and does not need to be solved. This is the next logical step. Resisting emotion and the other mental trappings that take place assume that emotion is a problem and does need to be solved. When you remind yourself that everything you feel is okay and your emotion is never a problem tension falls away. Please remember, I am saying that the emotion is never a problem, I am not saying that a life situation is never a problem, it is very easy to get this confused. I have had many clients say to me that whatever is going on in work or at home IS a problem. My response is that the feelings their intelligent body is sending are never a problem their job is to guide you back to your true self so that you can take action in the real world in order to solve the perceived problem. Anger with a work colleague is your intelligent body inviting you to act authentically, do what is right for you. The anger is never a problem and therefore should never be resisted or buried. The work colleague stealing your sandwiches from the office fridge is a problem and your true self wants you to take some constructive action.

3. Thinking will make you feel worse and you'll end up slipping down the spectrum towards Low Consciousness. When you think in an attempt to solve your emotion you are effectively getting in the way of your natural flow. Like the Weeble you will wobble more.

4. As your emotion is guiding you to back to your true self, allow yourself to be, to flow as best you can. You may know deep down where you are being nudged, what you really want in a given situation. If not, don't worry, it will come. There will be countless examples in your life where you have been in a state of high consciousness and flowed with effortless ease without the intervention of excessive thought. Sometimes it can be very difficult to work out whether we need to act or whether we just need to allow ourselves to feel and that is Okay, we can allow ourselves to not know. We are going to talk much more about this as we progress through the book. Acting authentically and constructively on emotion is one of the hardest things to do, especially when we live in a world that generally encourages either burying emotion or acting in a destructive way. The most important thing to begin with is allowing yourself to feel.

## Where Do Insight and Wisdom Come From?

If you were to stop and think about it, when do you get your best ideas? When do you get your inspiration? Despite sounding somewhat lighthearted, it is extremely common for many people to get their best ideas, their inspiration when in the shower, driving their car, riding their bike, out on a walk, or working on their garden. Why? Because this is often when the mind is clear, when there is an absence of mental churning.

I get my best ideas when talking to clients. My head is clear, I am in alignment with my true self and I'm flowing. I am not thinking about what I'm saying, I'm just opening my mouth and allowing whatever comes out to flow. I never get ideas to solve problems when I am stuck in my head or trying to think. I trust that my true self will always have an answer, it will always have a solution and I need to get out of the way and trust that the solution will flow.

When we feel overwhelmed or really stuck, we tend to increase our level of thinking. It's as if we have a baseline level of thinking that's always going on in the background, then when we are faced with a difficulty, a challenge, or a problem, we automatically look to thinking to solve our problem. So we venture north into our head in the hope that the solution will be found there. As we've already discussed, following this path tends to leave us spiraling down towards

Low Consciousness, a cluttered mind, and significant discomfort, even body symptoms.

So what we need to do is the opposite. Stay in your body and trust that your true self will deliver a solution if one is needed. The way I like to think of this is like the popular trust exercise that is often included in workshops and training programs. If you're not familiar with this exercise, the idea is that either with a partner or a small group, you are invited to close your eyes and fall backwards—falling backwards being completely unnatural and something your body will not want to do. You are placing all your trust in your partner or group to catch you, the idea being that you completely let go and trust. I like to think that my true self is a bit like the group. It has the answers, it will guide me, I just have to let go, stop struggling and resisting and trying to figure it out by thinking and simply allow my true self to catch me. When I do this and allow myself to fall back and trust my true self, my wisdom and insight flow with effortless ease. Access to our intuition and inner wisdom is heightened when we are connected to our true self and aligned with our core frequency and not thinking. The idea that thinking will solve the problem is completely misguided—it doesn't.

## Is There Ever a Good Time to Think?

In short, yes. If we can allow ourselves to detach our identity from our thinking brain and see thinking as a tool to use when appropriate it makes life a little easier and a lot more comfortable. Rather than the default assumption that we have to analyze and rationalize everything, we can simply apply our thinking skills when appropriate. We are always going to think and we could argue the ability to think is a wonderful gift. What is important is knowing when to think and when to get out of the way and let your true self guide you. Make sure that when you are thinking it is an activity you are consciously engaged in for a purpose. Too frequently we are engaged in one activity while thinking about several others, ruminating and churning, getting lost in thoughts that are not related to what we are doing right now. So when is the best time to think?

- When you are emotionally "clear"—this means there is a minimal amount of negative emotion present in your mind and body. Remember that our thinking is affected by our emotion, so as best you can make your decisions and do your thinking when your mind and body are clear and you feel connected to your true self. When you drop down the consciousness spectrum your thinking will be negatively affected. As you learn to detect this you will remember to avoid thinking, remembering that the thinking is not true, it is just a reflection of your state of consciousness at that moment in time.

- When the subject matter has nothing to do with your emotional experience. Examples are strategizing, or any form of intellectual assignment, such as solving a problem on your computer, or writing a report at work.
- When we have recognized and acknowledged our emotion and we want to engage in the most appropriate course of action. An example could be that you feel frustration and know that it relates to the performance of a member of staff at work. You know that acting or reacting impulsively will lead to you behaving in a destructive manner, so you engage in a small amount of very directed conscious thinking to identify some potential courses of action. You then allow yourself to be guided by intuition, wisdom, and insight when selecting the right course of action for you.
- Planning. This often requires a combination of thinking, insight, and feeling. For example, if you are planning a vacation, there may be various factors you want to consider, attaining a good balance of thinking and feeling can be extremely useful.

Thinking is an integral part of life, but it is important to understand its nature and cause as well as the role it plays in our identity, the creation of our reality. Despite discussing thinking in some detail, our aim is not to get in at the coal face and try to manipulate thinking, because, as we have seen that only leads to more thinking and a disconnection from the self.

Now that we have covered the basic ideas and theory, we have laid the foundations on which to build your recovery. In Part II we will be taking the theory from Part I, directing it and applying it to symptoms of fatigue, pain, and even anxiety and depression.

# PART II

## The Road To Recovery

## Let's Get Started

I N PART I WE EXPLORED THE THEORY AND PRINCIPLES THAT form the foundation of Energy-flow Coaching™. In Part II, we are going to get practical. This part is a guidebook to help you understand the connection between your emotions, your sense of identity, and your health and vitality. Our aim is to move towards an inside-out perspective, meaning that we are stepping into empowerment and assuming that we have the resources we need to experience health and wellness. All of the exercises in Part II could be seen as props, they are there merely to facilitate a realignment with your true self, so that you feel your emotions and intuitions. This means that there is not a set sequence of techniques that you must adhere to. The exercises are designed to give you a gentle nudge to get you back in alignment, they are not meant to be exercises that you think you have to do every day in a regimented way. I would also encourage you to be playful with the exercises you chose to do. There is no right and wrong and even though you may have a tendency to want to do it absolutely right, as best you can resist this urge and allow yourself to have the experience of the exercises. Be curious about what you experience, don't dictate what you must experience before taking part.

Your starting point is to get accustomed to how it feels to be in your body in the present moment. We are not looking to force ourselves to be constantly present in each moment because that simply isn't natural. However, being stuck in our thinking brain can become something of a full-time occupation, so redressing the balance is important. As you develop open awareness it will be easier to spend a little less time stuck in your thinking brain and a little more time in your body. The benefit of this is it enables you to detect the feedback from your intelligent-body—feelings and intuitions.

Probably the simplest way of getting into the body is by placing attention on your breathing and encouraging it to flow naturally. This is not like meditating where you take 20 minutes per day to place your attention on your breathing. This is an exercise where you learn to direct your attention to your breathing as you are going about your daily life. Whether you are washing dishes, writing emails, taking a shower, walking in the park, watching TV, or other daily activities, you can allow yourself to momentarily direct a portion of your attention to your breathing without stopping what you are doing. You can continue writing an email or reading this book and still take an aspect of your attention and nudge yourself towards your natural rhythmic breathing flow. This need only take a few seconds or minutes at most, however, regular practice will yield results and you will soon find your breathing is slower, deeper, and more regular. When you begin this practice you will probably find that your breathing patterns are staggered, interrupted, and inconsistent. This means you probably breathe high in your chest, frequently stop breathing, and hold your breath. Dysfunctional breathing patterns often arise from a body that is trapped in a state of stress and can become a habit in and of themselves. A cycle then begins whereby the disrupted breathing that originated from a body in a state of ongoing stress, if continued, then acts as feedback to the body that something is not right, which keeps the body in a state of stress.

Please remember that this is just a foundational piece, natural rhythmic breathing is not meant to alleviate symptoms, it is merely laying the groundwork. Our natural breathing pattern is a smooth and steady cycle in and out and the aim of this exercise is to offer a nudge back to that natural cycle.

1. Drop your attention down into your body—around the middle of your torso.
2. Direct your attention to your breathing.
3. Breathe from your stomach as long as it feels comfortable— so as you breathe in and out, allow your stomach to expand and contract rather than your chest go up and down.
4. You might want to try breathing in for a count of three

and out for a count of five—you may need to build up to this. If it feels uncomfortable do not force it.

5. As you practice this you will notice that your out-breath will feel very comfortable, being slightly slower than your in-breath.

6. The most important element is attaining and maintaining a continuous, steady cycle of in and out without force. This simply means no pausing on the in or out breath, maintain a continuous flow of breathing.

7. The aim is deeper, slower, more conscious natural breathing.

8. Once you have your comfortable cycle of breathing, there is an extra piece to the exercise that you could play with. Allow yourself to place your attention in each of your senses in turn; starting with your eyes, be aware of everything you can see, notice how much more you see as you open your awareness to what comes into your visual field. Then move to your ears, open up to everything you can hear all around; do sounds appear louder, do you find that you can hear more than you might expect? Then shift your attention to your nose and what you can smell; pause a moment and notice how you feel as you smell. Finally your proprioceptive sense, what you can feel through touch—this could be your back against the car or the wind on your face. Just be aware, be curious of everything that comes into your senses, then finish by allowing yourself to be aware of any emotional feelings or intuitions that may present themselves.

When to do the exercise:

Set an intention that you are going to return to your natural flow of breathing. Then, as you catch your attention throughout the day bring it back just for a moment and go through the steps above. This is not a process to alleviate symptoms and it is not a process that you need to focus all your attention on. This is about developing a habit of optimal breathing and being more body aware. You will probably find that your body feels more comfortable and flowing as you reacquaint yourself with your natural flow of breath.

CHAPTER 7

# Symptoms Are Solutions

I N OUR KEY PRINCIPLES CHAPTER, WE OFFERED A NEW WAY to look at symptoms, particularly medically unexplained symptoms, depression, and anxiety. Adopting a slightly metaphorical perspective, I suggested that symptoms are purposeful messengers, a tap on the shoulder from an unhappy body, if you will. Just as we are alerted to a stone in our shoe through the messenger of pain in our foot that occurs right here right now; medically unexplained symptoms of pain and fatigue, as well as anxiety and depression, are trying to get our attention right now. They are trying to alert us, tapping us on the shoulder and offering an opinion about the nature of our interaction with our environment right now. They are telling us that our true self has become trapped or buried in this moment.

I know that notion might seem a little simplistic and that surely we need to undergo some sort of deep analysis to investigate the nature of symptoms. However, as this is a guide book, we need to adopt a pragmatic approach, we need to figure out a way of understanding what is happening inside us in order that we can take appropriate steps. Our aim is to quickly figure out what we can do and what we can't do.

For the most part, we tend to look at symptoms as just being a natural consequence of being ill. This perspective is common sense when looking at conditions such as the common cold or a case of the flu, where a pathogen has entered our body taken hold, and as our immune system fights off the virus a series of symptoms are produced. If we have flu we expect our symptoms to last for several days maybe even weeks. We don't look at each symptom as some sort of communication or messenger, we just expect the symptoms to be there for a period of time and we also expect them to gradually diminish over time. The only remedial action we take is to rest and perhaps take some over-the-counter medication to alleviate the symptoms, the same as we would if we had twisted an ankle while on a country walk. We experience a symptom of pain, which tells us that there is some damage. The pain symptoms are likely to present themselves for a few days. We rest, take anti-inflammatory medication, and wait for the symptoms to abate and the ankle to heal.

However, it is worth bearing in mind that the symptoms that are presenting themselves in this moment are still telling us something about what is happening in the body right now. In the case of flu antibodies, white blood cells and other processes kick into action to defeat the invading pathogen. The symptoms we experience are the result of the immune system trying to remove the virus. We also know that a pathogen can be present in the body without any symptoms presenting themselves—it is only when the infection multiplies causing damage to cells that symptoms manifest. One of the reasons the infection multiples is because the body is already in a state of stress, which could mean that emotion is blocked. Whether you exhibit symptoms of a cold or flu virus and the length of time you have those symptoms are both directly affected by the extent to which your body is in a state of stress.

When we look at the case of the twisted ankle, even though the primary cause is in the past (the forest walk) the symptoms you would experience in this moment are feedback that the ankle is still damaged. The pain presents itself as feedback to direct your behavior to minimize further damage. Looking at all symptoms as feedback of sorts is the first step to understanding what to do, what action to take.

So are medically unexplained symptoms and conditions different and how are they solutions? We have established that the body has a natural self-healing, self-correcting mechanism and as long as conditions in the body allow for it, self-healing occurs. What is also important to establish is whether the cause of symptoms is still present; if cause is still present, symptoms will persist, if the cause is no longer present and conditions are conducive within the body, healing takes place. Medically unexplained conditions of fatigue and pain are likely to have a number of causes that act something like a combination lock. One of the most significant causes is emotional energy that gets blocked and imbalanced. While the roots of this pattern lie in childhood in most instances, it is the ongoing nature of emotional imbalance and blockage that leads to persistent symptoms.

Let's look at that in a little more detail. From the moment we are born our true self communicates to us through our intelligent-body via emotions, intuitions, and inner knowing. As we move through life, coping with the trials, tribulations, and bumps in the road can be difficult. Overwhelming emotions are often suppressed or blocked in order for us to focus on getting through a difficult situation. This burying or suppressing does not happen consciously on purpose, it happens unconsciously in order to get by, cope, and survive. Behavioral habits can form quite quickly, so if we have unconsciously pushed our emotion to one side in a particular situation in life and we have come out the other end of that situation, this pattern of pushing emotion to one side sticks with us. I see this over and over again with clients that I work with. As young people, they have either been brought up in a family environment that does not really allow for emotional acknowledgment and expression, or they have experienced one or a number of traumatic situations that could range from the seemingly mild to the very severe. What follows is often a lifelong pattern of emotional suppression.

Time, life contexts, circumstances, and people can all change, but the pattern of burying emotion becomes ingrained and resides outside of conscious awareness. If you are experiencing chronic fatigue or pain the circumstances in your life may be very different now as compared to when the symptoms first presented themselves to you. The key point being that it is not the external factors that really matter it is what has happened to the emotional feelings that your intelligent body has sent. Over a period of time blocking and shoving down ultimately results in a rewiring of neural pathways or overactivity in the brain and irregularities in the body's systems. It is almost as if our true self has to communicate to us through our intelligent-body and if emotions and intuitions are not getting through it turns up the volume in an attempt to get our attention.

Once this overactivity or rewiring has been activated it only requires a small emotional trigger to result in the presence of symptoms. This is why symptoms are the solutions, because despite their discomfort they are still just trying to get your attention to have you align with your true self by paying attention to your intelligent-body. Underneath those symptoms are emotions and intuitions that you are not feeling when they arise. Without doubt there will be emotions that you do feel, but in certain circumstances feelings will be bypassed and emotions will move straight to symptoms (remember we mentioned earlier in the book that emotions and feelings are slightly different and involve different structures in the brain). It's almost as if the symptoms are trying to get your attention to guide you back to your true self. If you suffer from chronic fatigue, fibromyalgia, anxiety, or depression there is a very good chance that you either don't really feel much emotion, or your emotional experience is distorted and very different from how it used to be when you didn't experience symptoms.

> From a young age, Simon witnessed his father behave in an outwardly aggressive manner. Simon had no recollection of suffering abuse at the hands of his father, he just remembered his father's anger, which would be triggered quite easily. As an empath, Simon would feel deeply uncomfortable when his father would display his anger and rage and he would do all he could to get away from the situation, usually running to his bedroom and locking the door. "I guess at some level I just decided that I was never going to be like that, I was never going to allow myself to be like my father, his behavior was so destructive. I wasn't aware of it at the time, but looking back I can see that it got to a point and I simply wouldn't let myself have anger, so I buried it, I wasn't going to be destructive like my father." This pattern developed over a period of time, but once in place it became part of who Simon thought he was. He believed that he was a person who simply didn't experience anger.
>
> While at a conscious level Simon wasn't aware of anger, his intelligent-body was still sending anger but it was getting squashed down in Simon's emotional stress bucket. He began to experience chronic pain symptoms in his neck, shoulders and back and fatigue that would render him useless. Medical investigation revealed no structural damage so he sought a variety of alternative treatments including acupuncture and osteopathy, which only provided temporary relief from the pain symptoms. As a police officer, Simon's work often required significant physical exertion. He was part of a squad that was involved in breaking down doors and making arrests. As he talked about

*this aspect of his job he expressed his amazement that symptoms didn't present themselves when he focused and channeled his energy and aggression into a forceful procedure. As we began working together his awareness developed of how he had buried his anger and learned to define himself as a person who didn't experience anger. He could see that it was this ongoing burying of anger that was resulting in the chronic pain symptoms he was experiencing. The fluctuations in his symptoms were alerting him to when anger was simultaneously triggered and buried. As he worked through the process he was able to translate his symptoms into emotions, which were predominantly anger based emotions. He learned to feel and constructively express and act on the anger, recognizing it as a communication inviting him to act authentically at a given time in a given situation.*

## Looking at Symptoms as Blocked Energy

So if the message or communication from symptoms is that there is a blocking or imbalance or emotional or intuitive energy right now, what steps do we need to take to redress this balance and allow our energy to flow? The first step is to increase your awareness of when your symptoms are presenting themselves. Whether it be Chronic Fatigue Syndrome, ME, Post Viral Fatigue, Adrenal Fatigue, Irritable Bowel Syndrome, Depression or Anxiety, symptoms almost always fluctuate. In the majority of cases there are symptoms that seem to be ever present, we could call these the baseline level of symptoms. Then there are the symptoms that seem to increase and decrease, these are the fluctuating symptoms. To begin with I would like you to focus on the fluctuating symptoms.

If you think about the last few days or week, can you remember how symptom levels have changed? If you can't, you might want to take a day or so and allow yourself to simply be aware of how your symptoms change. A significant proportion of my clients with chronic fatigue and pain symptoms have told me that their symptoms are always the same and never change. After several days of practising open awareness and allowing themselves to pay attention to symptom levels, they've noticed that symptoms do vary and fluctuate. In fact, many clients have told me that symptoms seem more intense or severe at the start of the process, primarily because they have done their best to ignore or tune out. Symptoms have appeared to be ever present, but this is largely because of the significant efforts made to push them aside.

Symptoms could be aches, pains, fatigue, brain fog or other cognitive problems, stomach and bowel discomfort, anxiety, sudden changes of mood. A fluctuation could mean that you notice changes in symptom levels over the last hour, or it could be that you notice a fairly sudden increase in symptoms over five or ten minutes. It could even be that you have noticed symptoms gradually increase over the course of a morning or afternoon. The key point is that you need to allow your awareness to develop for the changes and fluctuations in symptoms, especially when you notice that symptoms are increasing, because symptoms increases are an indication that your true self is seeking to get your attention. Being aware of symptom increases is one thing, knowing what to do is something else, and that is what we are moving on to next.

To begin with, let's keep things simple; let's assume that when there is an increase in symptoms, some low vibrational emotions are lurking underneath that lie outside of your conscious awareness. Just as a reminder, the low vibrational emotions most likely to trigger symptoms are, anger, frustration, fear, guilt, boredom, and shame, or some combination of these.

Try this process as soon as you notice your symptoms increase:

1. Stop what you are doing, bring all your energy and attention into the present moment and place your attention on the outside of your head. What I mean is that I want you to resist getting pulled into internal chatter and instead notice what is going on around you. What are you doing, who are you with?

2. Make a change to your approach or change what you are doing, or how you are expressing something. A change can be as simple as turning off your TV; changing the direction of a conversation; changing your physical location; saying "no" rather than "yes." It will all depend on what is happening right now. The clue is that when you get symptoms your true self is not happy in that moment. Something is blocked, either some emotions such as anger or boredom, or you are not being true to yourself.

3. Notice how you feel and what happens to your symptom level as you change your actions or approach.
4. If there is no change in symptoms, change something else that you are doing or saying and notice the impact on symptoms.

The purpose of this exercise is for you to begin noticing how your intelligent-body responds to life as it is unfolding now. Emotions are the energetic feedback regarding your interaction with your environment right in this moment. This concept can take some getting used to, as we are so accustomed to analyzing what is going on and looking for complicated explanations from the past or searching for solutions in the future. As a first step, we want to look at the simple things that are happening right now, right under your nose.

The principal point of this exercise is to practice being observational. The art of being observational is a skill. From when we are very young we have a tendency to draw conclusions about what we observe and assume that we are simply observing. When young children are asked to note down their observations and conclusions at school there is rarely a difference between the two. The key to success is to imagine that you are an outsider looking in, just watching and making notes.

An example of being observational could be: "It's 2:30 p.m., I'm sitting in Starbucks next to the door talking to my friend Sandra who is seated opposite me. Starbucks is full and the noise level is quite high. Sandra is talking about her job. There is a high turnover of customers and the door is opening and closing frequently."

So being observational is being objective, like the outsider looking in. It is devoid of subjective interpretation, opinion, and belief. When completing the exercise above you don't necessarily need a great deal of detail, but the more detail you have the greater the opportunity you have to understand what is going on emotionally underneath the symptoms.

Let's look in more detail at our Starbucks example. If we imagine that this is a real example for you, and you have noticed that symptoms have increased around 2:30, what might your low vibrational emotions be trying to communicate? Let's look at some potentials:

1. It could be that you have an appointment at 3 p.m. and Sandra is talking a great deal but you are concerned about saying you need

to leave. Your true self needs to get moving because it's a 30-minute drive to your appointment but you are not telling Sandra that you have to go, because you don't want to offend her. The problem is that when symptoms start to increase you then focus on symptoms and start thinking about being late and the long drive across town. As a result fear is produced as you get stuck in the "what if" pattern of, "what if I'm late and miss my appointment?" and, "what if my symptoms are too bad for me to be able to drive?" As these thoughts enter your head and fear is triggered, symptoms begin to increase. If you were to realize that the initial symptom onset was because the emotions were guiding you back to what you needed to do, i.e. tell Sandra that you need to leave, then go; when you act on that, your symptoms would reduce.

2. As Sandra is talking the door is opening and closing with people coming in and out of the shop. It's winter and each time the door opens a slug of cold air shoots into the shop. This frequent opening and closing is distracting and frustrating. However, you act as if everything is okay and pretend that you are following what Sandra is saying even though you are not. As symptoms begin to increase you begin to think about the implications of having symptoms, how they are likely to affect you now and for the rest of the day. The fear increases leading to an increase in symptoms. If you quickly notice that you are not happy with the cold draft and distracting comings and goings of customers, you can tell Sandra that you need to move to a different location within the shop. When you find a new table in a quieter corner your symptoms abate.

3. Sandra has a tendency to be a little bossy and try to get people to do things for her. Rather than asking you, in a roundabout sort of way she is telling you that you are going to do a favor for her and you find yourself agreeing even though this is not something you want to do, or even can do. This example is difficult to detect at the time, but as Sandra is a friend you meet a lot, the chances of this kind of example is likely to repeat itself. Learning from this experience is important.

4. You introduced Sandra to her boyfriend, Tom; he's one of your oldest and closest friends. As you are talking, Sandra is complaining about Tom and running him down. Much of what she is saying is not

true, as far as you are concerned. You just sit and listen and nod occasionally. Deep down there is anger because your true self wants to disagree with Sandra and remind her of Tom's good qualities. However, as you allow yourself to deviate from your true self, symptoms tap you on the shoulder.

This list of examples is not exhaustive but offers some potential ideas based on real-life examples. If you were sat in Starbucks and noticed symptoms increasing, I would suggest a trip to the bathroom to practice your observational skills and align yourself with your true self so you can figure out a course of constructive action.

There is no right or wrong action, this is a process of trial and error. The journey we are taking is one where we are looking to shed old conditioned patterns of behaving that are not aligned with your true self. You'll probably find that your tendency is to want to check that what you feel and what you do is "normal," what other people would do, or is what you "should" do. In aligning with your true self, you are effectively letting go of the need to do or say "the right thing," or what other people would do. You know when you have done the "right" thing for you, because your symptoms will reduce, and you will feel connected.

## Let Your Feelings Flow, Without Resistance

When our body and brain trigger negative emotions such as fear, anger, and guilt, the same areas of the brain are activated as when physical pain is experienced. When we experience a physical pain we tend to wince, flinch and do all we can to get away from the source of the pain and even disassociate from the pain itself. Disassociating is literally separating or putting distance between you and the pain. If you were to cut your hand with a kitchen knife and begin to disassociate, you would look at your hand as if it were someone else's hand, having it seem a long way from you would diminish the pain. Conversely, associating with the pain, "Oh my God, that's my hand, and it's damaged and hurting," and fear plays a significant role in the experience of pain. Despite it subjective nature, like all emotions, pain serves a useful purpose of quickly alerting you to something that could cause structural damage to your body.

Emotional "pain" is a little more complex because there is not always an obvious course of available action. However, the survival instinct is still evident and seeks to escape the uncomfortable emotion. We unconsciously disassociate from overwhelming emotions as a way of protecting ourselves. It's almost as if there is a part of us that figures out that if there is nothing that can be done about these overwhelming emotions that are flooding through the body and brain, we are better off splitting apart from them. This seems almost obvious when looking at children who are dependent on adults and are unable to control their immediate environment or situation. The problem that arises from disassociating from our emotion is that get backed-up in our stress bucket and a habit of disassociating is formed, which ultimately leads to the rewiring of neural pathways and symptoms.

Given that our natural tendency is to both feel our physical feelings and also resist feelings when they are uncomfortable and overwhelming, how do we navigate our way through this seemingly strange and complex world of feeling? We have already covered getting reacquainted with being a little more present in our bodies, the next step is to acknowledge everything we feel, accept it and allow it, without resistance, question or judgment. Let's make no mistake, allowing our emotion to flow without resistance requires a little focused attention, because of our natural instinctive tendency to resist and disassociate from discomfort. However, the payoff is significant.

As you look to develop your ability to allow your feelings and emotions to flow, it can be useful to have some insight into what may prevent your emotional-flow, what gets in the way. Here are the common patterns to be aware of.

PHYSICAL RESISTANCE: when our body sends low vibrational feelings the chain reaction of responses tends to follow a path whereby we tense up, stop breathing or change our breathing pattern, and attempt to push the feelings away. This is resistance in action and it can lead to a buildup of tension that lingers beneath your awareness radar. This tension signals to your brain that something is not quite right, so it remains in alert mode. Your body can remain in this state for hours after some emotion has been triggered if you allow it. You've probably had the experience of driving somewhere and either been late or stuck in heavy traffic, and because of the unconscious meaning you place on being or stuck in traffic or late your intelligent body responds by sending some emotions of agitation, annoyance, and frustration. You don't want to feel or experience this so you either consciously or unconsciously resist. The tension sits in your body and you arrive at your destination, which could be your office or some other place of work. Your behavior is affected by the tension and you are curt or sharp with colleagues or customers. A couple of phone calls later and your agitation breeds agitation and the tension in your body builds. You have slipped down the consciousness spectrum and your perceptions are more negative and hostile as a result. All the while you are ignoring it and pushing it aside in an attempt to get on with your day. By lunchtime you either have a headache or some other pain and fatigue-type symptom.

COGNITIVE RESISTANCE: How often have you found yourself saying, either to yourself or to others, "Is it normal to feel this?" or "Do other people feel this? I shouldn't feel like this, I should feel differently to this. I don't want to feel like this, I don't want to be the sort of person that feels like this." "If I allow myself to feel these emotions, it means . . ." Cognitive resistance of our emotional-flow comes in the form of comparisons of how we "should" feel, judgments about our feelings and whether we should have those feelings, and the attribution of meaning to those feelings—i.e., what it says or means about you for having those feelings. When your thinking centers activate with the presence of emotion the purpose is to identify an appropriate course of constructive action. However, what usually results is an excess of cognitive resistance trying to solve, analyze or find meaning in the feelings and emotions. All this thinking makes us feel worse, takes us away from identifying an appropriate course of action, and tends to prolong the negative feelings we are experiencing as we slip into lower consciousness.

These patterns get in the way of us feeling our feelings, so taking a little time to shift the way we respond will prove to be extremely useful. Changing this habit to one of acceptance rather than resistance requires intention and a little focus. Use the exercises you have been practicing up to this point of allowing your breathing to flow and reminding yourself that everything you feel is ok.

Another important piece at this point is that despite your desire to do so, you never have to justify, defend, or explain what you feel or why you feel what you feel to yourself or to anyone else. Like much of what is talked about in this book, it may seem like common sense, yet our tendency is to defend or justify both our feelings and any actions associated with those feelings. The reason is that we want to feel normal; we want to feel connected, not isolated. If other people feel what we feel then it's okay for us to feel like this, isn't it? It seems a plausible and sensible argument; however, when we walk that path of justifying and defending our feelings the result is resistance and blocking of our feelings and a denial of ourselves.

Your feelings and emotions are your truth in the moment that they arise. They are a reflection of who you are in that moment, but they are not the totality of you. What you feel today maybe different from what you feel tomorrow, so your feelings don't mean anything about you. They are your feedback, your navigational tool in that moment, bringing you back to your true self, your core essence. All you need to do is let yourself experience the physical sensations associated with feelings and notice how they change and move as you breathe and place your attention on them.

Many people feel anger as tightness in the chest, coupled with heaviness or tightness in other areas such as the forehead, neck, shoulders or even down the arms. The sensations will move and flow as you notice them and place your attention on them. Remember, just like the rumbling sensations associated with hunger, your emotional feelings are simply guiding you.

*Sally found it very difficult to say "no" and she always found herself justifying her feelings or defending her feelings when dealing with colleagues at work. She invariably got roped into doing things that she didn't really want to do, and if she did find a way of saying "no," she would spend long periods doubting and trying to justify her decisions and this would leave her feeling drained and emotionally depleted.*

*Tom, who shared the office with Sally, would always dump extra work on Sally. He wasn't consciously trying to get her to do the extras, but as she invariably said "yes," it had become the office pattern.*

*Sally said that if she didn't say "yes," she'd feel guilty. She'd never paused to feel into the guilt or where it came from so simply avoided it by saying "yes" every time Tom asked her to do something, or gave a five-minute explanation about her feelings in an attempt to justify herself and her decisions.*

*When Sally was presented with the idea of pausing first,*

*feeling into her core and then deciding what she wanted to do, rather than impulsively saying "yes," things began to change for her. To begin with, she found that she wanted to say "no" much more than she had before. She also found that as she practiced conscious breathing and staying present in her body in the now, it was not only easier to say "no" when it felt right, the guilt from saying "no" seemed to evaporate.*

*She practiced saying no without justifying her feelings and it felt great for her. Over time the pattern in the office began to change. Tom made fewer and fewer unreasonable requests and took on more responsibility. Interestingly, their working relationship improved. The deep-seated frustration and resentment that Sally was bottling up disappeared because she was now acting in alignment with her true self.*

## Acting on Emotions

The next step from accepting and acknowledging our feeling states is to take constructive action on them when appropriate and necessary. Continuing our theme that our emotion is guiding us back to home-base, inviting us to be our true selves in this current moment, there will be times that our emotional feedback is inviting us to take some action. We don't need to get caught up in trying to figure out exactly what the emotion is, whether it be anger, fear, frustration, annoyance, because often we are experiencing an amalgamation of emotions. All we need to be aware of is the level of emotional discomfort we are experiencing.

Emotion is often perceived negatively because of the actions people take in response to their emotion. Aggressive behavior is often seen as an anger problem. I would suggest that it is a behavioral problem not an emotional problem. Why? Because our emotion is never a problem, in the same way as our feeling of hunger is never a problem. If you're at the pizza parlor and you punch someone in the face and then run off with their pizza because you are famished, I don't imagine that anyone is going to blame your hunger.

Impulse, reactive and destructive behaviors are what give emotion a bad name. An interesting observation is that when your intelligent body sends a low vibrational feeling and you react to that feeling in an impulsive manner, it sends a signal that your intelligent body to produces more. For example, if you body were to send you the emotion of fear, there is a chance that your breathing will become shallower and move to be higher in your chest, your blood will be diverted away from your core towards your muscles. If you breathe in a shallow manner and start running, i.e. acting as if you are in fear, your body will respond by sending more fear. The same is true for anger; if you act in an aggressive manner, or even think about acting in an aggressive manner, you will notice that the amount of anger you feel in your body increases at that moment. The same pattern is evident with laughter; once you start laughing you tend to find more and more things will trigger laughter, so it takes less to make you laugh once you have started. This can be why once you "get the giggles" it's very hard to stop.

Let's look at what constructive action means in more detail. Rather than suggest that something "makes" you angry, simply recognize that you are experiencing anger at a particular moment in time, acknowledge and accept the feelings and sensations that are evident in your body. When we suggest that our emotional state is triggered by something outside of us, we remove our opportunity to take any action; we become helpless and hopeless. Remember that your emotion is never a problem and never needs to be solved; it is guiding you back to yourself and inviting you to act authentically, or in alignment with your true self at this moment in this situation. It is not about the other person, your emotion is about you; it is your opportunity to be true to yourself. If you don't take this opportunity there is a very good chance that your intelligent-body will send more anger or symptoms.

Pausing, breathing, and practicing constructive behavior in response to uncomfortable emotion is critical to enable emotion to flow, as opposed to seeing an amplification of that emotion. When you pause and breathe it far easier to act constructively rather than reacting destructively. Often when people feel anger there is an unconscious desire to enact revenge, however small, because anger frequently stems from hurt. This is how arguments start: "you hurt me, now I'm going to hurt you." Of course, you are not consciously thinking this, but your instinctive reptilian-brain wants to lash out. It's difficult to admit to this because we want to think of ourselves as nice, civilized people, and of course we are. We have that opportunity to shift away from those reptilian-brain urges into higher consciousness and take constructive action.

Let's look at the steps we need to take to ensure our actions are constructive and in our highest and best interest. Our actions always need to be a reflection of our true self in that moment, so we need to act from our core not from our mind trying to think about what we "should" do. We do want to be aware of what lies in our wake, the impact of our actions, however, ideally you want to avoid compromising your true self.

Can you think about the last time you felt the emotion of anger? As you do, picture the situation in your mind and feel the physical sensations in your body. As you reflect on that situation in your memory, what does your true self want you to do, to happen instead of what you are currently experiencing or witnessing? As you allow yourself to feel into that idea, can you get a sense of the most constructive action? To really simplify, we could suggest that you are currently experiencing A and your true self wants to be experiencing B, what's the best and most constructive way of getting there. Not long after my second daughter was born, my eldest daughter developed a cold and was waking up around 5:30am coughing and sneezing. She'd come in to see my wife and I and we'd comfort her and take her back to bed. After several days her cold had vanished but her pattern of waking at 5:30am and coming into our bedroom remained. Up to that point she tended to sleep through until 7:30am, which was ideal given that we had a new baby who was up in the night. After several days of being woken up at 5:30am after already having been woken by a new baby, my intelligent body started to send hints of frustration. I was working in management consulting at the time so had to get to work and be on top of my game, so I was concerned that my tiredness level would impact my ability to perform at my best. I could sense the reactive part of me wanted to just be firm with my eldest daughter and tell her in no uncertain terms to get back to bed at 5:30am. However, my true self sensed that this would probably result in feelings of guilt and was unlikely to yield the result that I wanted. My agitated frustration wanted me to find some way of getting a little more sleep, so how could I help my eldest daughter get back to her pattern of staying in bed until 7:30? It occurred to me that, despite being winter, there was a certain amount of light that would be visible from streetlights. My daughter had a very thin blind on her bedroom window and light from outside could be visible when she woke. I decided that a constructive action on my frustration was to go out, buy a blackout blind and fit it on her window. Luckily this did the trick, my daughter stopped coming into our bedroom at 5:30am and resumed her pattern of sleeping until 7:30. When we can figure out what we want to be experiencing and then how to get there in a constructive way, we are acting authentically on our emotional feedback. If I had decided that "good parents" didn't have anger about their children, I would have suppressed my true feelings and ironically this would have exacerbated my feelings of tiredness, or facilitated their development into something groggier or headaches.

Your emotion is never really about other people, it comes from inside you and is a nudge to get you back into alignment with your true self. If you can't work out or identify what you want to do in that moment, allow yourself to be okay with that, and have the intention that you will learn from what is happening and you will find an answer. This intention is important, it presupposes that you will find a solution and future solutions will emerge, and therefore it begins to shift your vibration and frequency in a more positive direction. If the emotional feeling is important it will come back to give you another nudge. If it isn't, as long as you allow yourself to feel it without resistance, you will notice that the emotional discomfort will soon subside and you will return to your higher consciousness space.

## Fear: The Ghost in Our Machine

Fear is the primary lower vibrational energy state that affects us in a plethora of different ways. As a negative emotion, it has an enormous influence on our behavior, our thoughts, our decisions and life choices.

Surface-level fear is evident when we feel nervous, concerned, worried, scared, petrified, and other such sentiments. In a very simple way, we could entertain the idea that these surface level fears relate to the unknown or missing information. So if we look at a situation and identify the unknowns or missing bits, we'll understand the cause of the fear. From this perspective when we acquire the missing information the amount of fear emotion that you are experiencing reduces. Let's look at a very simple example; if I am going to take my driving test in two hours' time I feel nervous—a member of the family of fear emotions. Following this rationale that fear can be viewed as missing information, what is the missing information? Well, I don't know what the examiner will be like, I don't know what route he will take me on, I don't know if I'll remember everything I've learned, and ultimately I don't know whether I will pass (the degree of importance I place on passing also affects my fear level). When I get in the car and start driving the missing information becomes known and my nervousness diminishes. Of course, if I make a series of mistakes I may become more nervous, especially if I have decided that I have to pass. This notion leads us to the next piece.

At a deeper level, fear is more of a misalignment of beliefs, unconscious expectations, and actions. This is where the mind has taken over and is ruling, dictating our actions and behaviors, and we are not in alignment with our true self. It is unconsciously stipulating that certain things need to happen and we feel fear when we believe we will fall short of these mind-set expectations. When fear drives our decisions and actions it can remain under the surface, making it difficult to detect. However, it will present itself as agitation, anger, and even anxiety. So if you notice yourself displaying seemingly unexplainable agitation, anger and anxiety you may find that there is deep level fear present. Straightforward examples are when you notice that your decisions and actions are based in "shoulds" and "musts". These are conditioned patterns stored in the mind that do not represent your true self's opinion and desire.

At its core, fear is about separation. It's interesting that quantum science and new spirituality talk about us being connected, all being one. Yet our five sense experience of life is very different. We experience ourselves and each other as detached and separate. The more separate we feel the more fear is present, the more "connected" we feel the less fear we experience. Our aim is to feel connected and aligned with our true self. The more we foster that connection the less deep level fear we experience. When we are aligned we are not trying to match ourselves to the outside world, we are allowing ourselves to flow. When we don't have to match the world and its supposed expectations we don't feel separate and deep level fear does not govern us. Surface level fear will serve us to a degree. When there are unknowns it can be helpful if we are alert to them. The key to moving beyond deep level fear is trust of your true self.

## Processing Fear, Anger, and Guilt

The three significant negative emotions that can cause havoc when they are blocked within the cells of the body are anger, fear, and guilt.

As a general rule, this is the only time in this program that you will be invited to look back in time. Every other exercise is concerned with now and making changes in the now. The reason we want to look back in this exercise is purely for the learning opportunity, to see if we can identify patterns that need to be shifted.

1. Get three pieces of paper and a pen and allow yourself about half an hour to go through this exercise.

2. On the first piece of paper under the heading "Anger," draw a line in the center of the page from the top to the bottom.

3. On the left-hand side, write a list of everything you can think of that has triggered anger in you in the past as well as in the present. This can be people, situations, events, etc.

4. When you have finished writing your list take a look at it. Are there any patterns, specifically in relation to people and the way they have treated you? For example, have people taken advantage of you, been mean or nasty to you or treated you badly in some way?

5. Now, remember that our goal is to take constructive action regarding our emotions and in doing so learn to become true to ourselves. On the right-hand side of the page next to each entry on the right, write down what constructive action you would take now—the newly empowered version of you. Does it feel right?

6. Repeat this exercise with "Fear" on the second sheet of paper. And then "Guilt" on the third piece of paper.

7. If there are blanks, that's perfectly okay. The important part is that you are beginning to tune yourself into seeking authentic constructive action.

8. The next step is to identify those things that trigger anger, fear, and guilt that are still present in your life now. Make a commitment to yourself to address those areas with constructive action.

9. Once you have completed this exercise with anger, fear and guilt, rip up the pieces of paper and put them in the trash. The reason for this is that as we will discover later, everything we say, do and write has an energy. We need

to deal with practical sources or triggers of negative emotion in our lives, then we want to ensure that the energy of what is written does not stick around to "contaminate" our energetic environment.

## Clearing What You Don't Want (or Need)

As an extension of the previous exercise, we want to identify those things that are not serving you in your current life. There are always going to be things in life that we don't want to do or don't like; however, it is important that we remain consciously aware of what we are choosing to do, how we are choosing to spend our time and energy. When we have lots of things in our life that no longer serve or we simply don't want, the buildup of negative emotion fills our stress bucket. It's so easy to move through life with a tendency to continue doing things out of habit, unaware of the emotional toll or impact. We often find ourselves with our busy lives, moving from one task to the next without really feeling our emotion. It can be easy to get trapped in doing the same things over and over. As we embrace empowered living we are making conscious choices for everything that we have in our lives. This is all part of directing and creating your life, moving past the abject helplessness that can characterize a disempowered and symptomatic life.

We don't want to dwell on what we don't want and what we don't like; however, we need to give it sufficient short-term attention to help us move it through and to encourage ourselves to move toward what we wish to experience.

This is a simple exercise that will address those things that bother you at some level, trigger uncomfortable feelings, or things you would simply like to change or have be different. As you do this exercise reflect on the people in your life, the places you find yourself—including your home, and the activities that you engage in— including work and non-work.

1. Write a list of everything you would like to change in your life. This could be a problem or something you want to be different. It could be something that bothers you or something you don't like or don't want. It could be sources of negative emotion or something that just isn't right.

2. Write next to it what you want instead, the ideal or opposite, what you would see, feel or experience with the
change. What do you wish to experience instead?

3. Imagine the change has taken place—what does it feel
like, how is your life different? Take as long as you need on
this step to imagine the difference and feel it in your body.
Notice where you feel the feelings, and as you pay attention to those feelings what images, if any, come to mind?

4. Is there anything stopping you from making the change?
Any obstacle blocking you or any additional resource
that you need?

5. What's the first step that you need to take? When will you
take it?

This is a useful exercise to implement whenever you feel overwhelmed or when things seem to be going wrong or getting on top
of you. Revisit your original document to update as you implement
changes. It is important to write them down on paper or on your
computer. Attempting to work through it in your head simply won't
be effective.

## Fluid States: Shifting Deep-Level Emotions

Even though feeling states and emotions are our guides navigating
us through life, there are times when emotions are being presented
because of a previous situation and are continuing to impact us even
though we have moved on. It is as if these old emotions can become
stuck and solid, "crystallizing" in our energy fields and unconscious.
These emotions are deep-level emotions and they can keep us locked
in energy bonds with people, situations, and activities. When this
happens you will find yourself repeating patterns of behavior without knowing why and those patterns won't seem to relate to who you
are now. It's almost as if there is an old part of you that keeps coming
back to kick you in the butt.

Emotions and feeling states are never fixed and our aim through
the exercise so far has been to facilitate their flow. However, on those
occasions where you feel discomfort and you can't identify an appropriate course of action and this feeling can be traced back in time, you
might want to play with the exercise below.

1. Identify something you want to change; an uncomfortable feeling state that feels stuck and is limiting you in that it is preventing you from moving forward or taking action in life.

2. Spend a few minutes exploring any potential learning not yet acknowledged from these seemingly stuck states. Remember, you are the focus, it is not about other people or trying to change other people. Experiences we have are for us to learn from, we need to place our attention on what we can learn from situations in order to fully master being ourselves and honoring ourselves.

3. Set an intention that you wish to transmute these stuck feeling states. We are not going to define what they will transmute into, simply create an intention that they will transmute in order to better serve you moving forward.

4. Allow yourself to fully feel the feelings and sensations associated with this state. Imagine welcoming and blessing this feeling state.

5. Imagine this state becoming more fluid and flexible. Revisit your intention to allow this state to change and transmute in alignment with your highest and best interest.

6. Allow any images to flow. These many be abstract images of things flowing and moving. If there are no images do not attempt to create images.

7. Once you have set the intention let it go. Do not include a timescale or another emotional state that you want to experience. Simply bless the existing state, feel it, set the intention for it to energetically transmute, then let it go, set it free.

8. Notice what happens over the coming days and weeks.

CHAPTER 8

# Defining YOU!

*HONORING YOURSELF IS REALIZING AND MAXIMIZING YOUR POTENtial; unleashing all of who you really are, without question, without judgment, without limits. Fulfillment doesn't come through what you get in your life; it comes through living the unique experience and expression of yourself throughout your life.*

The purpose of your life is to experience yourself as fully and completely as you can. To step out into the world and feel and engage with life in every moment. We are all unique expressions of consciousness and experiencing our individuality is a key component of our well-being. In this chapter, we are going to explore the importance of being you and defining you. The more you are able to align with your true self, your core-frequency, the better your health and vitality and the more you experience peace of mind.

Even though most of the time we feel distinct and separate from others, at a deeper level we are connected. If you were to sit on a sandy beach and look out to sea on a windy day, you would observe a body of water, undulating, swaying, and expressing itself. Each distinct wave is a unique expression, individual yet connected to the whole. Could you stop for a moment and feel into the notion that everything is connected; the trees, flowers, even the people at work? If you have seen the movie, *The Matrix*, you might remember one of the final scenes where the character, Neo, is able to see the Matrix as lines of code all connected. What if there was something beyond our current level of perception that connected everything in our world? Even though our eyes and brains decode everything as being separate, what if at the unseen level we are all connected? As you imagine this now, how does it change the way you see the world? Feeling connected and at one with all life is a natural byproduct of being aligned with high vibrational consciousness. Meditators often experience a greater sense of oneness and connection as their brain hemispheres synchronize during meditation practice. The high vibrational experience of love facilitates a feeling of oneness. Conversely, low vibrational fear facilitates separation and isolation; the more fear you feel the more isolated and separate you feel. I'm sure you will have had times in your life where you have felt connected and other times where you have felt isolated. Crucially, when you feel isolated and separate it is not that this is "true"; it is an indication that you have slipped down the consciousness spectrum and out of alignment with your true self. Even if this seems alien to you at this stage, I would invite you to just entertain the possibility that you and all around you are intimately connected and the more you move back up the spectrum to higher vibrational consciousness the more you will experience a sense of connection.

With that said, this chapter is about defining you. Our aim is to move towards the experience of a deeper sense of oneness while retaining our unique individuality and expression. This is where developing awareness of ourselves through feeling become important. It can be easy to get caught up in other people's energy, or the energy of mass consciousness. This is when we loose sight of where other people end and we begin, what is them and what is you. If you are an empathic person you will probably have had this experience. Another common experience is taking on other people's opinions as if they are our own without realizing. Or when we go along with others, thinking it's what we want, but deep in our core it isn't; or when we look to put other people before ourselves, forgetting ourselves as if we are not important. When these things happen we become misaligned and out of sync with our true self.

## Who's the Judge?

Have you noticed how prevalent judging and judgments are? In truth, it's quite difficult to determine exactly what is a judgment and what is simply a decision. For our purposes we'll suggest a judgment is something with negative consequences. In order for us to make judgments, we have to believe that there is right and wrong, good and bad. While at some level there is value in retaining a moral framework that serves as something of a guidebook to life, these morals ideally need to be kept to very basic principles of how we behave in relation to others and the planet. The problem is that when we judge as either good or bad we are beginning to distort or manipulate reality. Our perceptions are being manipulated and we are imprinting meaning. We often focus on what should and shouldn't happen in life and how we should and shouldn't be; this is good that is bad.

This dualistic or polarized thinking is commonplace and is not restricted to judgments of good, bad, right and wrong. As I talked about the Key Principles chapter, I've noticed over the years in my practice that when I invite people to feel into some options for moving forward the tendency is to entertain only two possibilities. It's either, I can do this or not do it, or, I could do this or that (where this and that tend to be opposites). I have no idea why this dualistic thinking tends to be the norm, whether this is hardwired into the brain or simply a manifestation of cultural indoctrination. Either way, it's not something we are stuck with and is most certainly a practice we can move beyond for our own benefit.

As we move towards existing within the space of the expanded-self it becomes a little easier to recognize that right, wrong, good and bad are constructs that we imprint upon life. They serve us in some respects but work against us in many others. It can be far more useful to allow yourself to see life and events as experiences. It's not that option A is good and option B is bad, both options A and B give different experiences, neither are good nor bad, right nor wrong. Our tendency to hold onto ideas and expectations about future events results in us resisting what unfolds. If we are open to both A and B as possible outcomes we are more likely to be open to any learning and beneficial experiences that result. When we judge we resist and any potential learning that we could derive from a situation tends to get lost. For example, if you were faced with a situation at work and you judged and blamed a colleague for wrong-doing, then you'd get caught up in the emotion that arises from focusing externally and blaming. If this situation is somehow serving you, judgments would block that learning.

I would suggest that, as best you can, allow yourself to view everything that happens in a neutral way. If you were to stop for a moment and contemplate the future, you can imagine that there are an almost infinite number of potentials and possibilities for things that could happen, especially if we factor in little nuances that make each experience unique. Each one of these potentials and possibilities brings with it a different experience. That experience is neither good nor bad, right nor wrong, it is simply experience. I recognize that this may leave you feeling a little uncomfortable because surely there has to be a right or wrong; however, I am simply inviting you to entertain the notion that everything is simply experience at this stage, in order for you to FEEL what it is like when judgment is removed. If you can feel this you will be able to see the extent to which judgment blocks the flow of energy and can lead to all sorts of problems.

Try this exercise:

1. Spend one week noticing those situations and circumstances that don't turn out quite as your mind had planned.
2. When you begin to feel the discomfort within your body, pause, bring your attention fully into your body and breathe.
3. Remind yourself that everything that happens is okay; it is here to serve you, there is something to learn from it.
4. This is the key question: "How does this situation make me feel about me, about myself?" Note, this is a completely different question than "How does this make me feel?" We are not asking that question. We are asking "How does this make me feel about myself?" If you get an answer like, "I feel like I'm not good enough" or "I feel pretty worthless," these are the learning points. The next question is: What do you need to do differently in order to feel good enough? How can you treat yourself differently to feel worthy?
5. Notice what happens to the discomfort in your body.
6. Can you see what you can learn from this situation? If you cannot, simply set an intention that you are open to learning from this situation and that you will remain an open vessel to that learning. If nothing else, you are learning to be flexible and not get stuck in resisting situations and circumstances simply because they did not turn out like your mind had planned.

## Setting Boundaries

The subject of boundaries is fairly common in personal development and therapy and it principally involves creating a boundary between you and others to protect yourself. When you go out into the world and set your boundaries you will be standing-up for yourself, being assertive, protecting and defending yourself. While this perspective can be of value to some, the Energy-flow model comes from a slightly different perspective. Rather than have a focus on other people and protecting yourself against other them, our focus is on defining you, allowing yourself to flow and your energy to radiate. When we have a strong energy and weak boundaries we run the risk of losing ourselves, compromising ourselves, allowing others to take advantage of us or treat us unfairly. Crucially you'll know if someone is crossing your boundaries because you'll either experience an increase in body tension, emotions or symptoms.

These are the steps to follow when you are faced with "boundary crossers."

1. If you sense or feel that you are being unfairly treated take some constructive action to put a stop to or prevent that unfair treatment—this could be a friend who takes advantage of you, or a colleague who dumps extra work on you, etc.

2. When reviewing situations, remove any judgment from the situation and those involved. Everything we encounter in life can serve us in some way if we are open to learning from these life situations. When we judge we block learning; judgment anchors you or sticks you to something. When we remove judgment we open the doors to learning and our Energy-flow. This is not an easy concept to grasp as we spend so much time judging ourselves and others in subtle ways that we often don't realize.

3. Think for a moment about someone who has "made" you angry. Look at how you are judging the person and the situation. Allow yourself to step into a perceptual space where you can see that you have an opportunity to learn something about yourself from this situation. This could even be something like, "This person is giving me an

opportunity to build firmer boundaries to define myself more effectively."

4. When you make that switch from blaming them, or thinking of them as bad or evil for having treated you badly, and start to see that they have offered you a positive opportunity, you move out of the victim space and then you are able to make effective general changes in your life. It becomes easier to align your behavior with your true self because the need to enact revenge dissipates; you recognize that your emotion is about you not about them.

5. Review your life make a commitment that you are going to set clear boundaries for yourself.

## Putting Yourself First

You are the most important person in your life, without question. Your "job" as a human and spiritual being is to have the experience of being you, fully you, without compromise. Being you is not something you have to think about or seek advice about. Being you flows when you get out of your head and out of the way. When you unleash yourself you feel fully alive, attain peace of mind, and begin to feel your Energy-flow.

If you have ever been on an airplane, you will be familiar with the safety procedure that goes something like this:

*"In the event of a drop in cabin pressure, oxygen masks will fall down in front of you. Please make sure to fit your own mask first before helping the person next to you."*

This is "self-first" in action. In the context of being on a plane, it seems to make perfect sense that we need to make sure that we are okay before we attempt to help others. However, when it comes to our daily lives we often have a tendency to disregard this—often to our disadvantage.

One problem that often seems to get in the way is the notion that being you and putting yourself first is being selfish. Let's be clear at this point that selfish and self-first are very different. I'd like you to entertain the idea that selfish and selfless are at the opposite ends of a spectrum. Arguably these are the slightly dysfunctional opposites in that they both deny your true self. If you are being selfish you are denying your innate connection to everyone else and "all that is." You are blocking the flow of energy and the flow of life. Selfishness comes from a foundation of fear; what this essentially means is that if we were to strip away the surface layers and look at the underlying motivation and drive it would be deep level fear.

At the other end of the spectrum we have self-less. Being self-less denies the self and this leads us precariously into the victim-vortex. Self-less is where we fail to honor and respect ourselves and we put others before ourselves. Self-first lies in the middle of our spectrum or continuum and is our target.

Self-first is when your actions and words are aligned with your core, you are flowing through what you do and say and your decisions and behaviors are based on what feels right for you. You consider others and you are mindful of the impact of your words and actions on other people. You feel a connection with those around you and possibly the earth and consciousness. You have a deep desire to be of service and to help others when this flows from being true to yourself.

> *Josie took her teenage daughters to a friend's birthday party. Life had been hectic at home, and the opportunity to spend time, quality time with her daughters had gone begging in recent months. The party was the first opportunity for a while for her to enjoy being with them. Despite her good intentions, on arrival at her friend's house she slipped back into old habits and started to think about what she should do to help. Josie took their coats into the spare room then immediately went to the kitchen and started to help with drinks and snacks to make sure everyone was having a good time. As a sufferer of fibromyalgia, it didn't take long before the usual suspects of headache and neck pain started to rear themselves. Her first instinct was to just push through, but something inside wanted her to stop and take notice. She gave two glasses of cava to Bob and Sheila who had just arrived, then she went straight to the bathroom. As she looked at herself in the mirror it hit her. She had always had a tendency to put everyone else before herself, and she knew that deep down she wanted to be with her daughters, laughing and joking and connecting with them. Recognizing that her symptoms were a tap on her shoulder, she made the decision to change her course of action, rather*

*than rushing round helping out to try and make sure everyone else was having a good time, she started to dance and laugh with her daughters. Within about half an hour her entire experience had shifted. Her symptoms were gone, her mood had lifted and she was having a great time. They danced for hours at the party without any reoccurrence of Josie's symptoms. On the car journey home, Josie's daughters commented that they'd had the best time with their mother in a long time, and other party members commented how Josie had made such a contribution to the party atmosphere. So, despite not helping with drinks, by putting herself first, she was actually helping in a different, perhaps more profound way.*

Here are three questions for you to consider:

1. Do you tend to put other people's wishes before your own?
2. Do you go along with what other people want even if deep down you don't really want to?
3. Do you feel guilty if you take time, money, or energy for yourself?

If you answered "yes" to any of these questions, you are probably either confusing selfish and self-first, or you have fallen into the unwanted habit of behaving as if for some reason other people are more important than you. The way you feel about yourself reflects the way you behave and the extent to which you allow your true self to show itself.

Back to our questions:

For each question you answered "yes," we need to begin to turn this around so it becomes a "no."

Looking at questions 1 and 2, I suggest that you draw up a list of people who you tend to put before yourself or go along with; then pick one or two days where your focus will be to reverse this trend. This could be something as simple as telling a friend that you would like to go to the movies tonight rather than sit and drink in the same bar as you did last week. Or that you would like to try cooking a new recipe you have seen rather than go out for dinner. What would happen if you paid attention to your true self; can you imagine a scenario where you follow your truth or put your needs first? Imagine this with a positive outcome for yourself and allow yourself to feel good about it.

Here is a fun exercise you could try to support this; take your notebook and write down five complimentary things about yourself. This can be very difficult if you are used to feeling down about yourself, so you can ease yourself in with something like, "I allow myself to feel all my emotions, they are valid and worthwhile," or, "I am willing to change and learn new things." As you get used to the idea you can move on towards something like, "I am a very special person." Try to pick five compliments that are meaningful to you. Take this page and put it next to your computer, or stick it on your fridge where you'll see it. Then when you're alone, say your statements out loud, yes out loud, and notice what you feel as you do. Try it for a week and notice what happens.

Here is a final more structured exercise you might want to play with on how to begin living self-first.

1. Identify in your life where you sense you are putting other people before yourself, going along with the wishes of others and doing things out of obligation or because you think you "should," rather than because it really feels right for you.
2. How can you begin to make changes? Identify the first small step you can take and make a commitment to taking that step.
3. Once you have done that review how you feel? Then plan the next steps and make a commitment to putting those into practice.
4. You will find that most people in your life won't notice any dramatic change in your behavior by putting yourself first, primarily because if your nature is to help, you are not going to cease helping. Small changes at this level can make an enormous difference to your physical and emotional health.

Taking time for yourself and giving energy to yourself is an extremely important part of fully taking care of yourself.

## Stepping Into Your Truth: Be Who You Are

We all have the potential to "act" or to be very different depending on circumstances and mood, and in so doing still retain a thread of authenticity that runs through what we say and do. We want to avoid tightly defining ourselves, and ideally we want to remain sufficiently present in the now so that we can simply be curious about who we might be, allowing ourselves to be ever-aware of our feeling feedback. However, what often happens is that we deviate from who we really are. We hide ourselves or cover up for fear of being found out, or revealing how we really feel. Or we pretend in order to be liked and accepted or not upset others.

The most important factor in how we behave is that we are doing so because it feels right for us in that moment, rather than doing or saying things because we are motivated by what others might think of us. Let's look at an example: Most people have the capacity to go to a party and either sit quietly in the corner or circulate around in a gregarious manner. These two are potential aspects of you and there are many more. Despite the desire to want to tightly define oneself as either extrovert or introvert, in truth, most people have the capacity to be either and lie somewhere on what is a broad spectrum. The most important point is that whether you choose to sit quietly in the corner or dance on tables, you are doing so because you want to, you are expressing and experiencing who you are in that moment. If you are sitting quietly or dancing around because you are conscious of what others will think, or because you think you should, then you are compromising your true self. This is when emotions or symptoms present themselves to give you a gentle reminder that you are deviating from home-base.

Let's take a closer look at how we block ourselves and cover up who we really are; then how we can begin to change these patterns.

### Performing

When was the last time you felt more than minor apprehension about being with people or meeting people? Maybe you experienced full-blown symptoms of anxiety, fatigue, pain or stomach upset, before, during or after the occasion. If you think back now, were you aware of thinking about how you should be, what you should say, or how you were going to conduct yourself? If so, there was a very good chance that the cause of your symptoms was that you put on a mask and were "performing," seeking to portray an image in order to fit in, be liked, or accepted. We are performing when the motivation driving our behavior is how others perceive us. Our focus and energy are on the outside, almost like a spotlight shining back on us. It's as if we are projecting our consciousness into some imaginary person who is looking at us, evaluating and judging us. But because we never really know what people think or how they perceive and judge, we fill in the requisite details in our own heads, and these details tend to be negative. In a desperate attempt to alleviate the internal discomfort that arises from this pursuit, we compromise and alter ourselves by performing. Our unconscious hope is that by being liked and accepted we will feel better. Unfortunately, what actually happens is that by altering, compromising and suppressing ourselves we block our Energy-flow and greater discomfort and symptoms arise.

Then we're stuck in a self-evaluation mind-loop, where we assume we know what others think and feel, and then we change ourselves in order to meet the ideals we have created. When we are performing for others in this way our energy tends to be dispersed and focused on the reaction of people around us.

If you were to stop for a moment and think of a time when you knew you were performing or behaving in a way to be accepted or liked or to be entertaining, as you remember that experience now you will probably also remember that your energy was focused on those around you, scattered, dispersed and somewhat fractured. If you find a different memory, one where you were being yourself, authentic rather than performing, you may remember that at the time you were flowing from the inside-out, the result being you feel better, more solid, grounded and generally happier and healthier.

### Performing: The Solution

1. Remember a time when you were totally yourself, notice what you feel, see and hear inside yourself.
2. Then remember a time when you knew you were "performing," or wearing a mask; what do you feel, see, and hear now?

3. Can you notice what is different about the memories? Did you find that when performing or wearing a mask you had a tendency to mentally rehearse words or actions before responding? Were there differences in the way you felt? Did you find your energy was more dispersed and focused on others when wearing the mask, whereas it was more centered in your core when you were being true to yourself?

4. In those situations can you imagine how you would be different if you were more yourself—without necessarily exposing yourself to the extent that you feel uncomfortable or awkward, rather how would you feel if you were more authentically you?

5. Next time you notice that you are not truly being yourself or wearing the mask, pause, bring your attention back to your core and practice letting who you really are fully flow.

6. The idea of this process is simply to give you a license to fully be who you are at any given moment.

## Covering Up Your True Feelings

Living in a culture of conformity, where everyone wants to appear "normal," there can be a strong tendency to cover up how we really feel. This can be in the form of stuffing down true feelings, going along with what others think, say or want to do, or even by stepping out of integrity and saying things we don't really mean. I encounter this pattern frequently where clients ask me if they are "normal" to have certain feelings. In almost all instances they have decided that they are not normal and they use this as an opportunity to beat themselves up and suppresses their feelings and themselves.

As you might imagine, I invite them to see that the question is misguided. Our job of allowing everything we feel to be okay means we have no more need to ask the question of whether what we feel is normal. In order to answer the question we have to compare ourselves with others, and comparing ourselves with others requires mental work and involves resistance, neither of which are part of the Energy-flow process.

*Covering Up Your True Feelings: The Solution*

1. If you stop and think about it, do you cover up your true feelings with certain people or in certain situations? If so, when do these situations occur and who are the people involved? Write these down on paper or in your notebook.

2. As you look at what you have written, do you feel that there is a reason why you cover up your true feelings?

3. Can you take a moment and go through the situations or people you have listed and imagine scenarios where you could be more authentic about how you feel, in a constructive way?

4. I'm not suggesting that you need to be open about everything you think and feel when you interact with others. I am suggesting that you do not compromise how you feel or cover it up in order to try to affect how other people perceive you—and that means tell the truth when you need to tell the truth. Covering up takes an enormous amount of energy—so it is extremely stressful—and disconnects you from your true self.

5. When you feel comfortable imagine being more authentic, allow yourself to pick the right opportunities to begin to practice.

6. Continue to practice until your authenticity becomes more second nature to you.

*Managing Other People's Emotions*

Have you noticed that when other people feel a negative emotion you tense up? And, have you noticed that your level of discomfort is even greater if you think that their negative emotion is "caused" by you? As an empathic person you may experience this sort of thing on at least a weekly, if not daily basis. Because we want to move away from discomfort as quickly as possible, and we are often driven from the unconscious belief that the outside world causes all our emotion, we tend to try to "fix" the other person's emotion in order to escape our discomfort. The drive can be incredibly strong to want to make the other person happy, because if they are happy, you will feel happy too—that's the way the logic of it works.

What happens is that we alter ourselves to be liked, avoid conflict and try to ensure the other person is not experiencing negative emotion because of us. The problem is that when we change, when we compromise who we are, we put ourselves in a box, and we are treating ourselves as if we are not good enough, not worthy, and the result is that we feel not good enough at best and symptomatic at worst. What's interesting is that most of the time we believe that our feelings of low self-esteem or lack of self-worth arise because of what happens to us in life. While in fact it is because of the way we treat ourselves, the way we change ourselves to have others accept and approve of us.

What results is an ongoing cycle of seeking external approval, validation, and acceptance in order to feel better. However, in doing this you are treating yourself as if you are not good enough and other people are better or more important than you. The outcome is you begin to feel that other people are better or more important, or you feel low and not good enough. It can even be the case that you feel anger or resentment initially as you compromise yourself, which can turn into feelings and symptoms as the emotion gets pushed down inside.

In most cases the emotion of resentment arises when we compromise ourselves for others. Then we tend to blame them, as if they caused our resentment. In truth, the resentment comes from our intelligent body as a reminder that we have compromised ourselves by trying to please or manage someone else's emotions. Our aim is to switch our perception so we can see that our emotion is about us and the way we are interacting with life, rather than seeing it as being caused by other people.

### Managing Other People's Emotions: The Solution

1. Experiencing both high and low vibrational emotions is part of the human experience. It is important to recognize there is no inherent right or wrong in people's emotional experience; it just is. As we practice removing judgment from emotion it is helpful to recognize that it is perfectly okay for people to feel whatever they feel.

2. Allow people to have their emotions and remind yourself that it is not your responsibility to change their emotional state or experience, regardless of what triggered their emotional state. This is not to say that you shouldn't

help people. What I am suggesting is that you avoid compromising yourself by taking full responsibility for the
emotions other people feel.

3. Simply pause and breathe when you recognize that you
are about to take responsibility for changing other people's feelings. Wait, don't rush in and try to change their
emotional state, let them experience it. If something deep
in your core presents itself as a course of action, take it,
but only if it feels right in your core and you are not acting out of a compulsion to change their emotions.

4. As with the exercise above, it might be useful to write in
your notebook a list of people with whom you know you
have tended to compromise yourself in order to manage
their emotions.

5. Once you have your list allow yourself to imagine interacting with them while allowing them to experience all
their emotions. Imagine yourself breathing and feeling
your own emotions.

6. Take this and implement it in your life, remembering that
it is your actions in the world that make the difference.

A common pattern here is emotional manipulation. Stop and
think for a moment, is there anyone in your life who, for whatever
reason, you seem compelled to change his or her emotional state or
experience? Or maybe there is someone who tries to "makes you feel
guilty" a lot? If so, it may be that you are stuck in an energetic pattern
or dynamic and the person is unconsciously emotionally manipulating you. Remember, there is no judgment here; we are merely witnessing a pattern. I would suggest that their behavior is not helpful
for you or them, and you are enabling the pattern by acting on guilt
or the compulsion to change their negative emotion. Resist the compulsion and avoid getting trapped in your mind by staying present
in the moment and connecting with your true self and do what feels
right for you.

When to implement these patterns:

Work on one pattern at a time and give yourself as much time as you
need until you feel comfortable identifying and working with it. I

cannot give you an absolute timescale for how long to work with this series of exercises because effective implementation will vary from person to person. The most important aspect, to begin with, is to consciously play with the patterns and allow whatever you experience to be okay. Then as you move on to other exercises in the program, maintain the intention that you are going to practice being your authentic self and you can consciously go through the exercises above as and when needed. These patterns are likely to be among those in the program that will require repeated reading and repeated visits. Some patterns are harder to shift than others, but it really is worth the effort.

## Be Good to Yourself

When I immersed myself within the world of personal development and then spirituality the notion of "loving yourself" was ubiquitous. The assumption was that many of life's discomforts had their root in a lack of self-love. While this seemed like a reasonable notion, I was left thinking, "What on earth does that mean, and how exactly do I do it?" In fact, I wondered what I was currently doing that meant I wasn't loving myself. The self-love preachers didn't really seem to have an answer to that, certainly not an answer that satisfied me. So I was left to feel inside and try and figure it out by myself. Maybe that was what they meant all along.

Self-love is a little bit like happiness, it's not something you do, it's something that is reflected in and emerges from what you do. We all know what it feels like to experience love in its different forms. The love for our children is a different experience from the love for our spouse or partner, which is different from the love we feel for our parents, or our friends. Each of these is different from the love for our favorite sports team or rock band. But how is self-love different? What does self-love feel like? Do we feel anything? It's certainly different from all those other types of love that are reflected outside of us.

I'd like to suggest that self-love is something of a journey rather than a destination. As you put yourself first, trust yourself and allow all your feelings to flow through you without resistance or judgment, the sense of connection and alignment that will emerge we could call loving the self. What arises when we fail to put ourselves first, trust our feelings and act from our true self is that we feel off-kilter, we slip into our low-consciousness space. You'll know when you've arrived because you are likely to experience derogatory or negative thoughts about yourself. This internal dialogue of self-loathing is common-place among those with health challenges, and the answer does not lie in challenging those thoughts. As we have talked about through the book, thinking leads to more thinking, and as the cause of those thoughts of self-judgment, self-doubt, and self-flagellation arise in part from our own interactions with the world around us, it is these interactions that we need to change and rather than battling the thoughts in our head.

As you begin to be nicer to yourself and treat yourself with the same honor and respect as you do those whom you love, the next step is to open yourself and allow others to be good to you. It's all too common to be the one giving; giving of yourself in terms of time or energy. How often do you really allow yourself to receive and accept? Or do you typically prefer to give rather than receive, always feeling a little uncomfortable receiving from others? You may think that it's a good to be of service and of course it is. However, if you believe that you are unable to receive because it is your role to be of service then you are doing yourself a disservice. Too many people who are empathic resist receiving because they believe it causes guilt or other emotional discomfort. This discomfort comes from the mind not the true self. If you recognize this pattern in yourself, it is time for you to begin to open up to receiving without condition. It can be very difficult to love yourself if you don't allow others to love you. Learning to receive unconditionally is a step in the direction of receiving love.

1. Notice how you feel when others give to you—do you feel comfort or discomfort?
2. When opportunities arise to receive from others, pause, breathe and allow yourself to embrace the opportunity. Allow yourself to receive without having to justify why you are receiving, or to have to give anything in return. Simply allow yourself to receive.
3. Practice creating space for yourself to receive rather closing down opportunities.
4. As you allow others to show love to you, your ability to love yourself will develop.

## Bringing You All Together: Self-Integration

Most of us are familiar with the idea that there are parts of us that we don't like or wish had never existed. These are primarily aspects of ourselves, our personality, physical characteristics, or experiences that we try to deny the existence of or leave out in the cold, so to speak. However, there may be feelings associated or meanings attached to physical features that you have tried to push down or ostracize; integrating these feeling states and perceptions of identity can be important—it's all part of loving ourselves. Integrating the light and dark without any judgment of right or wrong, good or bad. You are one whole being, a flowing entity if you will. Allowing all aspects of yourself to co-exist in harmony reduces the chances of those isolated parts of you trying to sabotage you. Trying too hard to be one thing without really acknowledging the other aspects breaks you apart and fractures your energy. Like all things, when we resist, ostracize, block or push away we don't eliminate we just cause more internal suffering. In order to transmute or change the energetic pattern or nature of something, we can't leave it out in the cold, we first have to welcome it back into the house, so to speak. When we integrate all aspects of ourselves we become just a little bit more whole. The key to success here again is allowing. When you are aware of those things about yourself that you resist or lock away, simply allow them to be. Breathe and allow, then notice what happens. As you occupy your expanded space just observe what you feel and notice how it flows.

## Developing Self-Esteem

There is an enormous industry based on boosting your self-esteem, and as far as I can tell, no one that I have come across has highlighted this very simple yet very powerful fact: the way you feel about yourself is a direct result of the way you treat yourself—it's about you not the world around you. At one level this may sound obvious, while on another level it may sound ridiculous. If you truly believe that your low self-esteem is caused by the way you were treated as a child, or the way you are treated by family or co-workers, or neighbors, then you are stuck in a misguided paradigm. It is easy to believe that the way we feel about ourselves is the result of the way others treat us, and that there is nothing we can do about the way other people treat us. When we believe this, our focus remains on the external, what is going on outside and how this impacts us.

So what exactly do I mean when I say the way we feel about ourselves is a direct result of the way we treat ourselves? There are two key areas that we have to consider here, so let's address them one by one to make sure everything is clear as we look to make some changes for the better.

## Thinking Patterns

You're probably familiar with beating yourself up with your internal thoughts, focusing on failure, and thinking that everything is going to go wrong. This arises simply because a certain area of the brain becomes overactive when emotional energy and our true self is blocked or out of alignment. How does it feel when you know that what your head is saying is not actually real, it's simply the result of a chain reaction? Then allow yourself to gently go through our simple process. Here's a reminder:

1. Remind yourself that the words in your head are not true. They are simply the result of overactivity in that part of your brain triggered by an energy buildup or blockage.
2. Redirect (but don't force) your attention into your body and breathe.
3. Reflect on where you are and what you are doing; what might be blocked? Are you bored, angry, frustrated, or not being yourself somehow and trying to fit in or impress others?
4. Can you change something about what you are doing to let your energy flow?
5. Stay with your breathing and your body and focus on flowing and doing something that will trigger a flow of positive emotion for you.

## Interactions with Others

How many people do you interact with on a daily or weekly basis? The way you behave with others affects not only how they treat you, but how you feel about you. Let's look at an example here:

*John thought that people at work didn't really take him seriously. He thought that he was seen as something of a joker or even a clown. Colleagues tended to be given more responsibility on projects and he could see himself being somewhat left behind as others progressed and moved their careers forward. John was left feeling very unhappy with the situation at work and wondered whether he should quit and find a new job. The problem with this idea was that his self-esteem had hit rock bottom. He'd been on a couple of interviews for other jobs but was finding that he was struggling to get past a first interview stage.*

*The notion or idea of being a clown or a joker had been with him as long as his self-esteem problems had troubled him, as long as he could remember. He wasn't consciously thinking, "I'm going to be a clown at work," but he was aware that he found himself behaving like this. What John didn't realize was that he was deviating from his true self, and projecting a joker or clown persona was causing people to treat him like this, and, more importantly, it was the biggest factor in why he felt so bad about himself.*

*When presented with this knowledge, John was able to reconnect with his true self, begin to work on being himself—which took some practice, but was something he was able to master. When he was true to himself he found that his self-esteem began to improve, he felt more confident in himself, less hesitant, and more capable. What was truly amazing for John was that other people began to treat him differently. He could see that it wasn't that people had treated him like a clown and therefore he had felt like a clown, but people treated him like a clown because that was how he felt about himself, that was the vibration he radiated, and that was how he behaved.*

## Taking Back Ownership of You

*The less you feel in control of your own internal experience, the more you will try to control your external environment.*

When you feel stressed, insecure, low, numb, anxious, or uncomfortable, the unconscious part of you will want to do all it can to minimize an ongoing buildup of negative, low vibrational emotion or blocked energy. Your true self will detect that the current energy is getting stuck or blocked and in an attempt to reduce any further buildup or imbalance, your mind will seek to control and manipulate external events and people.

However, a vitally important fact of life is that we cannot control events and people. While we are continually exerting an energetic influence on everything around us, this is very different from trying to directly control situations, events, and people. When we attempt to control external events and people the result is a massive buildup of internal tension.

So what is the answer? Rather than seeking to manipulate external events, you need to begin to redirect your attention inward. We cannot control external events or the emotions that arise in the moment, but we can direct our intention, attention, words, actions, and behaviors. The more you can allow yourself recognize that what you feel is never a problem and never needs to be solved, the less you will focus on trying to control the external world. When you are stuck in a pattern of seeking to control it will be largely unconscious. You are likely to simply feel out of control of yourself and without much thought you will seek to manipulate external circumstances.

We could suggest that an aspect of life mastery comes when we can tolerate and allow our emotional discomfort, letting it flow without having to suppress or block it.

Redirecting attention inward and allowing is the first step. Then play with the process below if it appeals to you.

1. Take a pen and paper and sit quietly for 10 to 15 minutes. Review your current life and think about people and situations that you try to control or avoid—it could be that you want people to think as you think, or you think things have to be a certain way, or happen in a particular way. Write these down as a list.

2. Go though the list and imagine how you would be different or how you would approach things differently if you were able to completely release the need for control. Everything you feel is okay, never needs to be solved, life does not directly cause what you feel, it is your interaction with life that most impacts your feeling states. All you have to focus on is you; you don't have need to

concern yourself with what others do. Remember, you have the capacity and ability to deal with anything that happens by effectively processing your emotional energy—i.e., focusing on you and being true to yourself

3. Pick a manageable number of entries from your list, and take two days to have them as your focus. Notice when you are seeking to control future events or other people's thinking or behavior.

4. Bring your attention back into your own body, allow yourself to breathe consciously, lock your attention into your core, and feel yourself beginning to flow.

5. Focus on what action (or non-action) feels right in the moment, as you let go of the need to control others or events and allow yourself to focus on letting yourself really flow.

6. You may notice that you don't actually control anything externally; rather you hold ideas and expectations in your mind as to how you want things to be and you hold yourself in a constant state of tension hoping that these mental representations or constructs play out. If this is the case, you will need to practice, allowing everything to be okay. Stay rooted in the present and remind yourself of this "I can allow myself to feel everything without judgment or restriction; I can allow myself to act on how I feel, nothing can harm me or affect me unless I allow it."

## Act From Core, Not Compulsion

As we strive to act from our authentic true self, developing awareness of the internal "drive" behind our behavior can be of value. Underneath every action there is a drive or motivation, which frequently presents itself as a feeling state. The most obvious examples being the sensations of thirst or hunger. What's important to remember is that all behavior will be underpinned by motivation or drive and if we don't know what that is, we might find that we are being maneuvered by old habits, compulsions or knee jerk reactions. As you move through this process you are practicing open awareness, expanding your sense of self and becoming more conscious in your choice of words and actions. In walking this path, eliminating patterns that don't serve you will be important, and understanding the motivations and drives behind your actions and behaviors will be useful for you. One of the biggest "drivers" behind our behavior that can have a detrimental impact by taking us away from our true self is compulsion. Compulsion is that urge to do or say something, often without really knowing why. It's an impulse that arises from the desire to either alleviate or avoid internal discomfort.

I'm not looking to "pathologize" compulsion or suggest that acting compulsively is representative of a problem. It is something that we all do in day-to-day life at some level. I'm sure you can identify with the urge to have to answer a text message immediately. Or when a friend or family member expresses frustration or anger and you feel compelled to try and change their emotional state, compelled to solve the problem for them, or simply offer advice and guidance. When you are acting out of compulsion the result can often be an increase in symptoms or just a feeling of low mood, flatness or some self-flagellation. Compulsion grows from a foundation of fear—we may not feel that fear, but it's lurking underneath our actions. Our aim is to shine a spotlight on those actions, bringing them into conscious awareness so that we can make choices that are in alignment with how we feel right now, who we are today.

1. If you stop for a moment and reflect on the last few weeks or perhaps longer, can you identify any times, either in certain situations or with specific people, where you tend to act out of compulsion, where you act impulsively in order to alleviate some deep internal discomfort?

2. Get a paper and pen and write down these situations or people. I imagine that the situations and people are likely to involve family and work.

3. Our aim in each of these instances is to break free from the compulsion and to act in alignment with what feels right in the moment.

4. Identify one or two of the areas you would like to work with, then set an intention that when you are with those people or in those situations that you as best you will take a course of action that feels right for you.

5. When you are in the situation with the person or peo-

ple, as best you can remain present in the moment, allow yourself to be aware of how you feel—without analyzing yourself, simply by having an aspect of your focus or attention on how you feel in the present moment.

6. When you notice the urge to act out of compulsion, pause, breathe, and attune to your inner wisdom, then do what feels right for you. In some instances this may be easy and in others not. Allow yourself to be playful with it, again, there are not right and wrong outcomes, you are learning to trust your inner wisdom, your true self and base your actions and decisions from this wisdom. It may be to begin with you do nothing, you simply notice the compulsive urge and you allow yourself to feel the discomfort of not acting in alignment with that compulsion. The more you create the space for your true self to communicate the easier it will be to let it flow.

# CHAPTER 9

# Speak Your Truth, Not Theirs

IN MY EXPERIENCE OF WORKING WITH EMOTION, THERE ARE two very common ideas that I keep bumping into. The first, as we've covered earlier, is that emotion simply arises as a result of thinking and in order to control and conquer our emotion we must master our thoughts. The other common notion is that emotion is some pesky nuisance from the past that we need to talk about. Verbalizing our feelings is believed to somehow release us from the emotional captivity in which we are enslaved. However, by now you are beginning to integrate this new understanding of emotion as being a nonconscious process that is giving us gentle nudges in the present moment, encouraging us to act in alignment with our true selves. As we have talked about it is much more useful for us to look at emotion as a feedback mechanism helping us navigate through our day-to-day experience than something we just need to verbalize.

I'm not suggesting there is anything wrong with talking about emotions, I'm just suggesting that in many instances it is not vital, not crucial. Emotions are important navigators, but just as talking about being hungry and wanting food doesn't fill you up, talking about emotion often isn't sufficient to satisfy its purpose. That said, there are times when we do need to express something verbally. It may be that we don't need to talk directly about the fact that we are experiencing emotion but the presence of emotion in relation to a situation or issue makes talking about it difficult. Crucially there are steps and a structure that we can follow that will make expressing emotion verbally a little easier. Before we get onto that, there are few other important areas we need to cover.

## The Power of Conformity

Imagine this; you are invited to participate in a psychology experiment to measure visual perceptions. You arrive and are sat in among a group of six other people. You are then shown a piece of card (A) with a line on it. A second piece of card (B) is then shown to you with three lines of varying lengths, one of which is the same length as the line on the first card. The experimenter then asks the group which line from card (B) matches the length of line the on card (A). All six of the other group members are asked before you and they give what you think is the wrong answer. What do you do?

This was the exact experiment performed by social psychologist Solomon Asch in 1951. His intention was to measure conformity. In this experiment, he found that a third of people would go along with the erroneous answer given by the group rather than the right answer. While there were a number of criticisms aimed at the study, the primary ones being that the experimental subjects were all male, and conformity in 1950s America was considered an intrinsic part of everyday values, the study is extremely interesting and the phenomenon of conformity is one which we need to be mindful of. There is a seductive energy about fitting in, going along with the crowd.

Crowd psychology suggests that the energetic dynamic of a crowd or situation can be so powerful as to overpower our normal psychological tendencies or capacities, i.e. we tend to behave very differently. The usual expectation is that our behavior becomes more destructive as we are overtaken by the low vibrational energy and emotion. We act impulsively following the energy of the group and lose our ability to use our higher thinking abilities and make conscious choices as we engage in impulsive behavior. The majority of research and interest in crowd psychology and conformity is based on how base, vulgar, deranged, and violent people can be when in a crowd, displaying behavior they wouldn't under normal circumstances.

However, this is not exclusively the case. A powerful energy and frequency can raise or lower the vibration. Mass energy and consciousness goes beyond the group environment and has the capacity to raise the vibration. This is something people frequently experience at religious ceremonies, spiritual gatherings, and even music festivals and concerts. The collective energy and psyche has a significant impact that radiates outwards. Author Lynn McTaggart has worked with a number of academics on what she calls Peace Intention Experiments. In these experiments, she has demonstrated that a large number of meditators holding a specific intention can facilitate a reduction in fatalities in war-torn regions or lower crime rates. While these results may seem fantastical, they are merely examples that we are somehow connected and our frequency and vibration can impact and influence the world around us.

The point I am looking to make is that there are significant influencers that impact us every day. I frequently read on social media posts that more than ninety-five percent of our behavior is unconscious and arises as a result of our conditioning. Mainstream cognitive science would have us believe that we have almost no free will in our behavioral choices, so how can we possibly stand in our own truth? It may be that I'm an idealist, but despite having the odds stacked against us, I do believe that we can step into our own truth, speak from our heart and make decisions that are aligned with our true self, our core frequency.

The primary focus of this chapter is verbal communication. How important is it for us to talk about our feelings, when do we need to do it, and when don't we need to do it.

## Speaking Our Truth

There are two questions that we need to address in this section; first, when do we need to speak our truth? Second, when do we need to speak about our emotions? The answer to the first question is, always. Ideally, everything that comes out of your mouth resonates with who you are. This, however, does not mean that you have to blurt out everything that pops into your mind. If you're walking along the road with your partner and you walk past someone you perceive to be particularly attractive, you do not have to immediately tell your partner because that is your truth in that moment. Standing in your truth means that what does come out of your mouth comes from your true self, it resonates with your core frequency. The notion of resonating is important because you will know the feeling when you are speaking from your true self rather than speaking from your conditioned mind. The feeling is different so recognizing this is important. As a fun experiment, try this; say out loud, "I am a man," and notice how you feel, then say out loud, "I am a woman" and notice how you feel. There will be a difference in how these feel in your body, depending on whether you are a man or a woman; one will resonate as your truth and one will not.

Only you can answer the second question. If it feels appropriate for you to tell someone how you feel then I would encourage you to do so. In saying that, it is important that your intention is not for that person to have to change. Words and language are frequently going to be the first step in trying to effect change in the world around you, but when other people are involved it is important to have a plan B.

For example, if your housemate or someone you live with has a habit of leaving the milk out of the fridge after using it, my guess would be that the first thing you will do is invite them to put it back. Ideally, they will do the honorable thing and make this simple behavioral change. However, when it comes to situations that are more emotive or more significant than milk outside the fridge, we have to apply some principles to help us navigate to where we want to be.

It is important that we are able to express ourselves in a way that is constructive and authentic, while at the same time recognizing that words may not lead to a change in someone else's behavior. In fact, because so much of our behavior arises from unconscious pattern you are better off assuming that a person won't change even if they have good intentions.

To begin addressing this idea, I would invite you to feel into the notion of letting go of the need for other people to change. Here's a simple example; let's say you have a friend you meet for coffee a few times a month, and every time your friend arrives up to thirty minutes late despite being the one who suggests the time. Even though we have talked about the idea that our emotion comes from inside us and is guiding us back to acting from our core in this moment, it would be a safe bet to suggest that you might experience some frustration, especially if this happens every time. The first thing you are going to want to do is tell your friend that you are frustrated. If you suffer from a chronic fatigue or pain condition as we have outlined, small emotions can trigger big symptoms, so you may find yourself in Starbucks staring at your watch as symptoms increase.

Formulating what to say is important; however, in an example such as this it is probably important to let go of the need for your friend to change. There is a very good chance that this friend is late for everything. I'm not going to start making excuses for your tardy chum, but I would say that people tend to process time in very different ways. Some people seem to get lost in time and have a real problem keeping appointments, while others are able to process time in a very linear manner. The ones who get lost in time tend to find it difficult to process time and need to refer to a clock. These people can pop to the shop to buy a newspaper and come home two hours later having chatted to various people and totally lost track of time. The people who process time in a very linear way simply wouldn't do this. They would sense time and feel uncomfortable at the notion of being late.

I am digressing here, but the point I am looking to make is that it is important to feel and acknowledge your emotion, and you may want to express it. However, it is important that you let go of the need for your friend to change. When I say 'let go' I am not suggesting that you pretend that you are not frustrated waiting for thirty minutes each time, I'm suggesting you allow what is happening without resistance, and you allow your frustration to be present, then you decide what action you can take based on how you feel. You need to look to yourself at how you are going to change what you do given the circumstances are as they are. Of course, it might be the case that your friend takes note of your comments and makes a decision to change—if that happens, great. If not you might want to try arriving thirty minutes after the agreed time, not to spite your friend, rather to act on the fact that your intelligent-body consistently sends frustration at waiting for this friend. Another alternative could be that you take a book or do some emails during your thirty-minute wait.

In my practice over the years, I have encountered many people who avoid expressing themselves at all costs because of a belief that it will go wrong; it will lead to conflict, or upset. When we choose to talk to others about our emotions or emotive subjects it can be difficult, often because we anticipate a defensive response, an argument of some kind, or hurt feelings. In helping my clients navigate this tricky path, I thought it would be interesting and important to gather some data about my client's experiences where they had communicated feelings to someone, only for it to result in an argument or conflagration of some sort. What emerged were some very simple patterns; there were certain things that were said, and more importantly the way they were said, that almost always resulted in the conversation turning south.

I was curious what would happen if we mapped out these patterns, looked at the opposite, and put those patterns into practice. This is what we found.

## The Experience of Language

Before we get into the patterns and steps you can take to make talking about emotional issues easier without the collateral damage that is so often incurred, let's take a very quick look at the impact language can have on our experience.

If you're game, and you're not sitting in a crowded coffee shop reading this book, can you say these following sentences out loud. While you do that place your attention in your body and notice what you feel.

*"I will have a great time with my friends."*
*"I can't have a great time with my friends"*
*"I did have a great time with my friends."*
*"I won't have a good time with my friends."*

Even if you can't read these words out loud and you can only read them in your head, you are likely to notice very different internal experiences with each of these sentences. I certainty did as I wrote them down, so I'm going to tell you what I experienced and you can compare it with yours. Just to emphasize there is absolutely no right or wrong with this, and if you feel almost nothing that's perfectly okay. If you are wondering why I asked you to say them out loud (or you could even write them yourself), it is because our intelligent-body often responds in a different way to thoughts as opposed to behavior. Speaking and writing are behaviors and will more than likely elicit a different feeling response than saying something in your head.

As I wrote the first sentence with "I will" I felt a sense of expansion and potential; I felt a tinge of excitement that manifest as a tingling sensation. I felt "floaty" and ready to go. As I wrote the second sentence, "I can't," I felt a feeling of contraction and constriction primarily in my chest and the back of my head. I felt rooted in my chair, heavy, and weighed down. As I read the third sentence, "I did," I felt feelings of nostalgia, like I was sitting back into my chair and smiling. What interested me was how different this feeling was from the first sentence. There was a real sense of looking back with contentment but there was none of the excitement, anticipation, and hope that accompanied the first. As I wrote the last, "I won't," I felt like a victim, like I was digging my heels in. I felt constricted all throughout my abdomen and the sense was I was restricting myself before I'd even given myself an opportunity; a door was closed and locked before I'd seen what was behind it.

That exercise took me about three minutes, and I can honestly say that I did it as I would want you to do it. I didn't spend time thinking about what I felt, I placed my attention in my body as I wrote and read the sentences and wrote down exactly what I felt without editing it. I am going to admit that it has been a long time since I have done a little exercise like that, and I was surprised at how significantly different my feelings were.

This very simple exercise gives us an insight into what we are going to cover in more detail in the last chapter, that is how we create our own experience of reality. Why is it that words create such strong internal feelings? The answer lies in frequency. We've been talking about our core frequency, a vibration that is truly us. When we use words that resonate with our core frequency we feel good—feelings in the body that are similar to expansion, lightness, pleasant tingling. When we use words that are misaligned with our true self that causes a harmonic dissonance that we feel most often as tightness, constriction, and other feelings of being trapped and restricted. There is a vibration and a frequency to language that impacts not only the person communicating but also the listener.

An example of the vibrational effect of language is described in the 2005 book, *The Hidden Messages*, written by Japanese scientist, Dr. Masaru Emoto. Drawing heavily on his own research, the author details the ability of water to absorb and be influenced by the vibrational impact of words, or more specifically the emotional content of words. In one simple experiment, he placed a glass of water over a piece of paper with the word "love" written on it and another over a piece of paper with the word "hate" written on it. Using high-speed photography, he analyzed the crystal structures formed in frozen water. His analysis revealed that coherently organized crystalline structures had formed over the word "love," while incoherent and disorganized crystalline structures had formed over the word "hate."

Emoto proposed that a property of water is to absorb and reflect a wide range of frequencies that reflect the environment.

What we are learning is that the language that we use is incredibly important. We know that we are receivers and transmitters of energy, and language is one of those mediums through which we transmit energy out into the world. When we are communicating through language and the content of what we are saying is emotional the energy becomes even more powerful.

## Setting the Scene

Moving back to our step by step process for verbally expressing ourselves in an effective and empowering manner, the first thing we need to do is set the scene. Introducing material that is emotive in some way can be very difficult and is often the reason why people fail to discuss how they really feel. There is a fear of getting it wrong or saying something in a clumsy way. Ideally we can take proactive action here and offer some form of preamble to set the scene. When conversations go wrong, it is often because the speaker goes straight to the point while feeling a significant amount of emotion, and the listener can feel somewhat hoodwinked. We do not want to be reactive from low consciousness, we want to be considered and compassionate in high consciousness. If you sense that you have tumbled down the consciousness spectrum wait before talking. When you are ready, here are a couple of examples of how you could set the scene:

*"I'd like to have a chat with you about something that is a little awkward for me to talk about, so I may be a little clumsy in what I'm saying. However, I'd be very grateful if you could hear me out."*

Or

*"There's something I need to talk about but I am finding it difficult to discuss so I'd really appreciate it if you would bear with me while we talk.,"*

Or

*" I really need to talk to you about something that is important for me. I'm not sure exactly how to word this so please bear with me."*

There are many variations that can be included here and finding the right words for you is important; remember that whatever you say needs to be a reflection of your true self; if my words don't resonate with you don't use them. Also keep in mind our inside-out approach;

rather than looking outside you for the solution, remember that you have the capacity within you to find the most appropriate words. There is no right or wrong way to express yourself; say what resonates with your true self and comes from a space of high consciousness. The idea here is that we are setting the scene and ideally preparing the person for a conversation that is important.

## Using Empowered Language

As we have already discussed, language is an energy that has an extremely powerful effect both on the speaker and the listener. The words we use create emotional experience for us as well as those we are speaking to. Words impact upon the way we perceive and conceive of reality, they influence the way we react and behave, they influence the direction of an interaction or relationship, and the course of our own lives.

With that in mind, our focus in this section is to speak with empowered language. This means using language that reflects that we are aligned with our true self, internally referenced and directing our decisions and choices regarding our behavior and actions. If we use language that assumes other people are responsible for what happens to us, we become disempowered. The energy of disempowerment manifests in statements such as "Why are you doing this to me," or, "Why are you making me do this," or "You are making me feel . . ." This energy and these types of statements often elicit a defensive response in the person we are talking to. Try saying these sentences out loud and notice what you feel in your body. Just like our earlier exercise, you'll probably notice some level of tension, discomfort or constriction.

When we use empowered language and assume responsibility for ourselves, we feel stronger, more confident, and in control of our immediate destiny and ourselves. When we use disempowered language and give away the responsibility for ourselves to others we feel weaker, more vulnerable, and more prone to resulting anger, frustration, and resentment. Because of the effect our language has on others, when we use disempowered language we are more prone to be treated unfairly or taken advantage of. When we use empowered language we command respect and we are more likely to be treated fairly. Empowered language is simply being clear about your feelings and intentions without questioning the validity or veracity of them.

## Integrity

When we stand in our truth and speak with integrity, the energy of our words is more powerful than when our words and actions are incongruous. Incongruity in this respect is saying one thing and doing another. It's amazingly easy to be incongruous because our egoic-mind tends to have one view of life while our intelligent body may have an entirely different view. We've all heard someone say how they "really don't care," only to exhibit signs and symptoms of stress and emotional discomfort. This person in all likelihood really thinks that they don't care, but their intelligent body has a very different view. The more we are in tune with our physical and emotional bodies, the less chance there is of mixed messages coursing through our mind body system.

Being in integrity with ourselves means only speaking our truth and following through with what we say. So, for example, if we tell a friend we are going to do something ideally we need to follow through and do it. I'm not saying there is not scope for changing one's decision based on different feelings, what I am saying is that it is important to create an energetic balance between our words and our actions. If we don't our words become weaker and others will feel it; they will feel the energy that you project. The cliché of "my word is my bond" has real meaning. When we are in integrity with ourselves, our words form a clear intention, which is followed with action resulting in a bond that extremely powerful.

## The Three Steps

Now we have set the scene we can look at the steps that can form the structure of how to talk to people in a way that allows you to express your true self without eliciting a defensive response.

1. Always talk about your feelings without blaming others for how you feel. It is very important that we avoid using the word "you," because this will more than likely evoke a defensive response.

For example, it is better to lead with, "I feel frustrated when . . ."; rather than, "You make me feel frustrated when you . . ."

2. Stick to facts. This step is much harder than it seems. Frequently we attribute meanings to what people have done or said, we draw conclusions about what people think or feel based on what they say. Often these assumptions are incorrect. When we are misaligned and in a state of low consciousness our tendency will be to perceive what we hear in a negative or destructive way. This is often when we react and lash out, moving further away from a solution. Our task is to make sure we identify the observable facts of a situation and speak about them without including other meaning-based comments and opinions. Meaning usually comes in the form of A = B or A leads to B; for example, you didn't say good morning when I arrived at the office so that means you don't like me. Not saying good morning = not liking. Drawing conclusions about other people's opinions, thoughts, feelings and beliefs based on their observable behavior is incredibly common (we all do it), and potentially damaging.

Example: *"I feel frustrated when the windows are left open and the cold air gets in."* Rather than, *"You've left the windows open again, you're so careless. If I really mattered to you, you would shut them."*

3. Identify and include a direction or solution where possible. This is much easier when in high consciousness because the desire to move towards a solution is in-built and will flow more easily. You will know if you are in low consciousness because your egoic-mind will want to fixate on what is going wrong and what it doesn't like. Recognizing this and moving away from those thoughts and placing your attention on what you want to experience, a solution, is the first step.

Whenever we talk about something that is emotional for us the person we are talking to will feel some of that energy. In order to minimize their discomfort and the chance of them responding negatively to the energy they pick up, we want to move towards a solution and away from the problem.

Example: *"I feel frustrated when the windows are open; would it be possible in future to close them so that I don't get cold. Thank you."*

Including others in this process can be useful especially if you can't think of a direction or solution.

Example: *"I know there's a solution to this, would you be able to help me find it"*

Or

*"I would really value your assistance in working through this towards an outcome that suits us both."*

Or

*"I can't think of a solution to this at the moment, but it would be great if we could talk about how to solve this issue."*

Or

*"I'm not sure which direction we need to move in, do you have any ideas."*

Without doubt, this will seem like absolute common sense, and it is. However, my little home research project showed that in most instances my clients were finding themselves waist deep in a shouting match when they were doing the exact opposite of what is outlined in the three steps.

While it seems easy because at one level it is obvious, it does take some practice. Like doing anything new, there is always a feeling of awkwardness. However, as you put this little process into action you will be amazed that you are able to effectively articulate your thoughts and feelings, and the response you get could be the exact opposite of what you expect.

I have had numerous clients report to me that their fear about having a particular conversation or discussion was that it would inevitably result in the other person being nasty or rejecting them in some way. When they plucked up their courage and implemented the process they were amazed at the outcome. You will notice that you will be able to speak your truth without upsetting people or finding yourself in arguments. Also, you will feel much more confident, and in control of yourself and the direction your life takes.

# CHAPTER 10

# There Are No Victims or Villains

WHEN I WAS A KID I'D GO TO MY GRANDPARENTS' HOUSE and watch Westerns with my grandfather. He'd seen them all, so he told me, but we loved watching those "cowboys and Indians" together. It was pretty clear in those movies who the good guys and bad guys were. Without doubt in my mind there were clear perpetrators of injustice, manipulators, victims, and heroes. Of course, Hollywood's job is to create drama in order to give us an emotional experience, tapping into our base instincts and primal emotions. But when we look at "real life" is it true that there are victims and villains, the downtrodden and the manipulators, or is there something else at play? Could it be that our dualistic polarized thinking ushers us towards categorizing experiences along perceptual guidelines; or could it be that we are so entrenched in outside-in thinking, where we categorically believe that the world happens to us?

In this chapter, we are going to entertain the idea that even though it often seems that we are victims and there are those who are manipulators, this is nothing more than an "energetic vortex" of low consciousness. It's as if we are playing a game, and sometimes we chose to play the role of victim and other times we choose to play the role of manipulator, or even rescuer. We don't consciously choose this; we are unconsciously driven by the old habits of who we think we are and the emotional pay-off arising from being a victim, a manipulator or a rescuer. But before we delve deeply into all that, let's take . . .

## A Brief Glimpse at the Meaning of Life

What is the meaning of life? What is the meaning of *your* life? Too off topic for this book? Possibly, but bear with me for a moment.

I'm pretty sure that when we go to school we don't address the big questions in life like, what does it all mean, who are we really, what are we doing here? Where are we going, and why? At the simplest level, we could suggest that the meaning of life is about having an experience of being human. To have the experience of being *you*, and live the full expression of you without the shackles and restrictions that often seem to temper our ability to experience ourselves. From the moment we are born we are impacted by the "energy" of life. The expectations and conditions we face take us away from our true self, and we end up being more of who we are not than who we really are. When our true self gets lost our intelligent body responds by sending us discomfort and symptoms. It's as if our body quite literally says "no" when we are not aligned with our true self.

We are sovereign beings, meaning we are unlimited, unbounded, unrestricted, unrestrained, unconditional, part of the whole, part of infinite consciousness. This connection that binds us together makes us equal. At the human level inequality is rampant, but at a higher level of consciousness we are all one where equality forms part of the fabric of reality. At this higher level of consciousness there are no victims and villains, there are only expressions of consciousness having subjective experiences in an infinite number of ways. Each and every one of us needs to stand in our own truth, to take responsibility for ourselves, realize that we are the reflections of each other, connected yet unique. We are part of the same whole, and there is part of us in everyone else. There is no better or worse, only different versions as we experience ourselves subjectively.

Why is this important? Seeing life and ourselves from a slightly different perspective can facilitate a deeper understanding of who we are. Witnessing from a higher perspective where we are part of a larger consciousness can help remove judgment, which reduces resistance and therefore suffering. Our experience as humans is separate and unique and I am not suggesting that we overlook this; quite the contrary, we should celebrate our idiosyncratic nature by allowing ourselves to align with our true self and flourish. But separation without the recognition of underlying connection is what leads to the experience of fear. When we are restricted and restrained we deviate from our true self and our vibration drops. When we see and feel ourselves as separate and not connected to the whole, we experience more low vibrational emotions of fear and anger—and this creates a cycle of more separation more fear. You may have heard the theory that there are two basic emotions: love and fear. I would suggest that there is high and low vibrational emotional energy that is all connected as part of the same spectrum. The more we see and experience ourselves as separate and not connected to "all that is," the more we experience low vibrational emotions. We also find ourselves becoming caught up in a low vibrational vortex that can leave us feeling like victims. The victim-manipulator-rescuer energy is extremely powerful and prevalent, and many of us have seen ourselves caught up in this vortex where, as we go through our interactions and encounters in life, we find ourselves playing out one of these roles, assuming this is reality, the single truth. However, that isn't the case it is merely a point of perception, a frequency that we have tuned into. Taking on the role of victim or manipulator creates inequality and drama. It is often when we get caught up in drama that we see these roles coming to the forefront.

Without doubt, you will know someone or maybe you are someone, who is always wrapped up in some drama or other. Drama can be something of an addiction in that there can seem like there is a strong gravitational pull towards situations that are dramatic. Why is this? As human beings we want emotional experience; having some emotion is better than no emotion. The significant amount of our emotional experience comes through interaction with other people, and so it follows that for the most part, drama involves other people.

## Life Is Such a Drama

Drama presents itself when we are craving some emotional experience regardless of its quality. When you find yourself getting into arguments with your spouse, partner, other family members or colleagues at work, there is a good chance that you are seeking the emotional experience that drama provides. You are not consciously seeking drama, you're unconsciously seeking an emotional experience. We love going to the movies because in that ninety minutes we are on a rollercoaster of emotion set against a backdrop of psychological safety. We can get pulled into the experience of the big screen and the emotion we feel is significant and real as we associate with characters portrayed in the films we watch. For those who suffer from chronic pain or fatigue conditions, it's not uncommon to experience increases in symptoms when watching movies. This, of course, begins to make sense as we entertain the idea that fluctuations in emotions, and spikes in the lower vibrational emotions, can lead to the onset of symptoms.

If you were to stop for a moment and think about your own life, how often find yourself in embroiled in drama? When the high energy of drama grabs us and pulls us in, our behavioral responses tend to be impulsive and reactive, they often come from low consciousness rather than high consciousness. Without doubt there will be someone in your life, be it a member of your family, a friend, or work colleague who's life seems like a perpetual episode in a TV drama series. Things go wrong, they've been wronged, you've been asked questions like, "Can you believe they did this," or "You wouldn't believe what happened." I'm not suggesting that drama is a "bad" thing, or that we need to avoid drama at all costs. What I am encouraging as part of this process is that you make conscious choices about what you do. Recognize the motivations behind your actions, and rather than being blindly pulled into reacting to high drama because the energy sucks you in. I would encourage you to pause and feel the flow of energy through your body, recognize that those involved may be addicted to the energetic allure of drama. Then you can decide whether you want to involve yourself or whether you would rather watch from behind a short wall, so to speak. If you step into drama at least recognize that this is what you are doing. In too many instances people fall into the trap of the notion of a single reality, the idea that this is just what happens, or more often, this is just what happens to me. Often polarized or dualistic thinking also kicks in in the form of, "I had no choice, what could I do, I am not going to do nothing so I did this." It's that notion that we are presented with two choices: either do nothing, or respond in "this" way. These are patterns we are looking to avoid because they lead to a buildup or peaks of toxic low vibrational emotion, and they keep us locked in that victim vortex.

When I began to see this pattern emerge in both my clients and my own life I could see the subtle yet significant impact it was having on perceptions of life, symptoms, and outcomes. There's a kind of insidious nature about being pulled into the victim vortex. Even though most of us would vociferously argue that we are not victims and do not act like victims, there is a huge amount of comfort gained from giving away responsibility for ourselves to others or to circumstance. I know that as a kid there would be times that I would sulk, pout, and protest that I had been wronged. The practice of being helpless, wallowing in self-pity in an attempt to manipulate others into feeling sorry for me or guilty about something they had or hadn't done became something of a habit. It was so much easier to feel sorry for myself, to sit in a hole of pity rather than figure out what I wanted. Now I'm not suggesting that this was a dominant factor in my childhood through to adult life, but it was a factor. But it was only when I saw it in others, that it really became evident the extent to which it was my reality too.

## Escaping the Victim-Vortex

*It is the prison without walls that we cannot escape. In order to experience emancipation, we need to first recognize that we are trapped. The cages that we build for ourselves through our beliefs and conditioning keep us locked in patterns of behaving and concepts of ourselves that prevent us from reaching our potential in every aspect of life.*

There is a well-known theory in psychology and cognitive science called confirmation bias; this is the tendency to seek out information that matches our pre-existing ideas, notions, and beliefs. So as human beings our tendency is to form unconscious beliefs and seek to ratify those beliefs through our perceptions and experiences. We interpret events from a perspective that confirms our existing ideas. When coupled with another psychological theory, cognitive dissonance, we can end up in a very interesting version of reality. Cognitive dissonance suggests that when we are faced with two opposing ideas, attitudes or beliefs we experience internal discomfort. As we know, our tendency as humans beings is to do what we can to move away from discomfort towards comfort, so we do what we can to remove the opposing ideas. If we are presented with evidence that runs counter to an existing belief our natural tendency will be a desire to hold onto that belief because we favor consistency over radically changing ideas and attitudes. We unconsciously attach our sense of identity to our ideas, attitudes, and beliefs so we fight to maintain them, pushing aside anything that may destabilize our sense of self.

Leon Festinger first investigated the idea of cognitive dissonance when researching cults. He found that if a cult believed the world was going to end with a flood and the flood didn't happen, rather than change their beliefs they tended to interpret events from the perspective that they had been right all along; they were spared by a merciful God who was rewarding them for their display of faith and good work. This offers a theoretical explanation of why people often behave in irrational or even maladaptive ways, because they are displaying cognitive dissonance and are seeking to maintain constancy and consistency.

Our senses are constantly bombarded with data every minute of every day. Our lives are busier, there are constant demands on our time and we are almost never in "off mode." We can't possibly take on board all of the information that is coming our way, so we tend to filter out huge chunks. I'm sure you've had the experience of buying a new car that you think you've rarely seen on the roads only to see the exact same car in the exact same color every time you step foot outside your house. This is an example of the way we unconsciously filter out "data" as it appears relevant to our experience of life. When we combine this with the theories of cognitive dissonance, and confirmation bias, we can begin to see that reality is not something that is fixed and objective, it really is open to interpretation. These are crucial theories that we need to understand if we are to effectively step out of and gain mastery over the victim-manipulator-rescuer vortex. Understanding that we are unconsciously manipulating our own perceptions of the world is so important.

From the conventional, we now need to move to the unconventional. Have you ever had the experience of walking into a room and feeling or sensing the energy? Or have you ever been to a party and you can sense the energy and atmosphere as you approach? I love it when I'm watching a sporting event and the commentator says how "You can cut the tension in the auditorium with a knife." We all know and sense that energy exists, an energy that we can't seem to explain, but somehow we feel it and it impacts our perceptions and behaviors.

Dr. Rollin McCraty and his team at the HeartMath Institute in California have conducted research to measure the electric and magnetic fields that are emitted by our brains and hearts. While my guess would be that these in no way fully explain the range of subtle energy that is experienced, it offers a starting point for some phenomena that as yet remain somewhat elusive to traditional and conventional methods of measurement. For our purposes. I am going to suggest that we are both transmitters and receivers of energy, electromagnetic energy as well as more subtle energies. So as we move through each and every moment of every day we are radiating and absorbing energy from the environment and other people. As we will go on to see in Chapter 11, the energy that we radiate plays a significant role in the creation of our experience. For this chapter, we are going to focus on moving beyond the victim-manipulator-rescuer vortex.

I use the word vortex in this context because I would like you to think of it as something of a whirlwind of your own creation. As we transmit energy and align ourselves using confirmation bias and cognitive dissonance, we create a vortex of energy. This vortex has the power to suck in energies that are related or connected somehow.

The way we can begin to recognize when we are pulled into the vortex is by the presence of drama, strong emotions or symptoms. The next step is to take responsibility for ourselves. We are not victims of circumstance we are creators of our own experience and we need to recognize this in order to take the appropriate steps into empowerment. You are not a victim, you are never a victim, you are a willing participant. Even though the conscious part of you will vociferously reject any notion that you may be contributing to what appears to be a negative experience, the irony being that it is this same aspect of you that labels the experience as negative, which contributes to its negativity affect. As you begin to implement the idea of allowing emotion without having to solve emotion, it will become easier to allow circumstances and accept that, even though consciously you may have no idea how or why you are going through this experience, at some level it serving you.

If you find that you are being manipulated, treated unfairly, taken advantage of in an obvious or insidious sort of way, you do need to stop or prevent that. I'm not suggesting this is easy; however when you remove judgment and you recognize that the emotions you are experiencing are about you and not about the other person or people involved and that they are not "doing something to you," it will be far easier to take constructive action and act from an aligned high consciousness space rather than reacting impulsively from a low consciousness space.

A tip is to remind yourself that this person is giving you an opportunity to step out of the victim vortex and into empowerment, and that if it wasn't this person in your life behaving in this way it would be someone else. Telling that person how you feel may work and is often the first step; however, as we discussed in the previous chapter it is always useful to have a plan B just in case articulating what you want doesn't pan out as desired.

What is critical is that you trust yourself, trust your feelings, and avoid rationalizing them away. Too frequently I have found that there is a tendency for the thinking brain to want to avoid the discomfort of dealing with a situation by finding all sorts of reasons for maintaining the current position. You might have a boss who treats you badly, but you find yourself searching for all the reasons why you shouldn't do anything about it, either because deep down he's a good guy, or because you fear you'll lose your job if you rock the apple cart.

This internal conflict of "heart" against "head" is as old as the ancient wisdom that recognized the enormous role the heart plays in trying to communicate the truth about who we are and our interaction with life. Making that decision to take that difficult step now and take some action to stop the unfair treatment will serve you enormously in the future. Failing to take action now will lead to more situations and circumstances like this, which will mean more drama, strong emotions, and symptoms.

The first step towards empowerment is to take responsibility for your words, actions, and thoughts. You are responsible for how you deal with your feelings and emotions—and we have seen how this affects your ongoing experience. This becomes a little easier if you can allow yourself to believe that everything that happens is happening *for* you rather than happening *to* you. This means that the people and situations that show up in your life are offering you an opportunity to experience something, or learn something; they are not sent to punish you. It is so easy to judge a situation as bad because it feels emotionally uncomfortable, or because our conscious-mind decided ahead of time that it wanted a different outcome. However, when you begin to open up to the possibility that there is something for you in all experiences, even if you don't yet know what that is, your resistance and low vibrational energy begin to shift.

Because you are the creator of your own emotional experience, the way you feel about yourself in a given situation is the true source of learning. This is very different from how something makes you feel, which is a common question asked in counseling; a question that assumes the external events are the cause of your emotion rather than your emotion coming from inside you. So if we look at the question how do you feel about *you* when something happens, we turn our attention inwards. For example, a work situation could leave you feeling angry and if you allow yourself to fall into the victim-vortex you would attribute that anger to a work colleague or boss who has made you angry. If we look at how you feel about you in that situation the answer could be that you feel useless or hopeless. This gives us something to work with. How we feel about ourselves is very often a reflection of how we are treating ourselves and the vibration we are radiating. So in this example, there is a strong likelihood that, at least some of the time, you are acting and behaving as if you are useless and hopeless, although this is likely to be outside of your conscious awareness. This is a concept and practice we will return to in more detail in Chapter 12, Life Design and Creation. As a starting point, allow yourself to recognize that you are responsible for yourself and how you interact with life, and whatever shows up in your life is partly your creation. Look at how you could change your approach, responses, words, behaviors, and interpretations in order to feel empowered, rather than seeing yourself as a victim.

By taking responsibility for our actions we impact our ongoing emotional experience. The irony is that if we try to control we become disempowered. There is an energy that encapsulates disempowerment and we are going to call this the victim-vortex. Our five-sense experience of reality can lead us to believe that life is happening *to* us, like we are victims of circumstance and there is nothing we can do. We have a tendency to blame other people and events and see everything as beyond our control. Our focus is external and how the external is impacting us. Every time we give responsibility for ourselves away to others, or blame others for how we feel or for our negative reactions, we are entering the victim-vortex. When we get sucked into the victim-vortex it can be difficult to pull ourselves out. We've all had the experience of feeling insecure or off-kilter and then either consciously or unconsciously try to manipulate or control events, circumstances or people. Tension builds inside and we feel even less able to deal with life so we seek to control events even more. We then get stuck in the victim-vortex. We believe life is happening to us and this causes us to feel negative emotions, so we try to control life circumstances in the hope of changing our emotional experience only to find that this causes more negative emotions because we are deviating from our true-selves.

When you have this knowledge and look in on the victim-vortex it seems obvious, but when you're in the midst of it, caught up and desperately fighting to feel better, it can seem like this is all real, this is all happening to you and there is nothing you can do to stop it.

What you will begin to notice is that by entering and occupying the victim-vortex will generate ongoing feelings of anger or hurt. It would be very easy to interpret these feelings as either emotions that are deep inside and need to come out, or as feelings created by the situation. Neither is strictly true. The feelings are created by what we do in that situation, how we interpret and interact with that situation now. Just because we have had a pattern of interpretation and action in the past does not mean that this is who we are or what we have to do in the future. If the way we act leads to ongoing negative feelings or symptoms then we know that it is not who we are, because those negative feelings are reminding us that we are deviating from our true self.

This pattern is something I am very familiar with because I had to work hard to move myself out of the victim-vortex. I can remember several occasions quite distinctly where I could feel an interpretation of a situation and see myself walking a path that kept me in the victim-vortex. As I entertained this potential course of action I could feel my body produce more feelings of hurt and anger. Then I could pull myself back to the starting point and entertain a different perspective or path, one where I was empowered, taking responsibility for my actions, assuming that the circumstances were happening for me rather than to me. I could sense what I wanted and what action to take that would be a reflection of my true self. As I entertained this idea I felt physically bigger, lighter, aligned, and clear.

It was like facing a fork in the road, I could quite literally come back to the starting point and take steps down either path, each time I could feel how my body responded. When I entertained the path that kept me locked in the victim-vortex my body would scream the feelings of hurt and anger. The feelings were not about something outside of me, they were not because of other people and caused by other people, these feelings were my body shouting at me to align with my core, to get out of the victim-vortex and to be my true self.

This was a deeply profound experience for me; I could see how I was literally creating my experience. The victim-vortex path had been my default so it took a little conscious effort on my behalf to pause and choose the empowered path that aligned with my true self. What I began to experience was a much more empowered and confident version of myself. I felt differently about myself and interestingly, I noticed that people responded to me in a different way. When I was radiating the vibration of disempowered "victim," my external experience reflected this back to me and this was how I was treated. The empowered experience was very different both internally and what I was witnessing externally. This was like a shard of light in a dark room, offering an insight into the role I was playing in the creation of my experience.

## Breaking the Rescuer-Helper Cycle

The other side of the victim vortex is the "rescuer-helper. As you might expect, the majority of our emotional experience arises as a result of interaction with other people, and there will be certain people in our lives, particular family members or close friends, who are the catalysts for the most amount of emotion we feel and experience. Because we are working with emotion and interpreting it as feedback, we could view these situations as a training ground for mastering the lessons that life throws at us. To help us move beyond the rescuer pattern we need to first understand how it manifests itself. Then we can begin to look at what needs to change.

### Type 1: The Good Listener

When it comes to verbal interactions there are levels of communication. At every level emotion will be evoked, from lighthearted chitchat to deep and meaningful conversations about the meaning of life. Communication is a highly emotional process for both speaker and listener. When speaking you will either be seeking to elicit an emotional response in your listener or you may anticipate an emotional experience yourself. You might be telling a story about some experience you had and want to share with others, or you might be sharing the office gossip. These all serve a purpose for us; they help us validate ourselves, foster a connection with others, and create a flow of energy between those we are communicating with. As a listener, you may have the experience of connecting with the person you are listening to, in which case you will again, experience a flow of emotion through you. If you are not a willing listener, if you are bored or become passive in the process of listening, your emotional experience is negative; frustration and boredom arise from the intelligent body and disrupt the system, which can cause feelings of fatigue and agitation.

As a "rescuer," you are likely to define yourself a nice person who is always there to help. You will have experienced positive feedback about being there for others, being easygoing and possibly a good person to talk to. Despite the fact that your nature or natural wiring results in you being a good person, there is a very good chance that the unconscious drive to maintain that identity and please others pushes you beyond alignment with your true self into the victim vortex. This means that there will be times when you over-ride the feedback from your true self in order to maintain the identity as a nice person. This is when you spend that extra time listening to your friend's problems, or you take that extra time on the phone to try and find a solution and offer guidance despite needing to deal with your own life in that moment.

There are two clear traps that you can fall into as a listener. The first is remaining passive in communication and allowing you to be burdened.

Here's an example of Pattern 1.

> Sandra had been experiencing a six-month period of bouts of extreme fatigue and muscle pain. She had blood tests but her doctor could offer no explanation as to the cause of her symptoms. She was offered painkillers and antidepressants. Sandra's best friend, Denise, had been experiencing problems at work and with her husband. Sandra thought of herself as a good listener and thought she really should be there for Denise—after all, Denise was there for her, wasn't she? Denise had the sort

*of boss who was only really interested in getting his job done. He hadn't received any training in how to manage people and it showed. He'd worked his way up through the ranks and was pretty good with numbers and figures but lacked the skills and desire to get the best out of the team he managed. The result was that there was a level of tension in the office that was often palpable. Arguments would ensue and problems were rarely dealt with and resolved in a constructive manner. This was coupled with the fact that Denise's boyfriend played pool for the local pub team and was spending an increasing number of evenings going to play other pubs' teams. Denise had never been one to focus on solving her problems and issues, but she liked to talk about them at length. She liked to lean on Sandra, though she was never aware that this was what she was doing. Denise knew if she spoke to Sandra she could offload and unburden, and Sandra would always make her feel better. The bad news for Sandra, however, was that she would find that speaking with Denise would always leave her feeling an increase in her symptoms, fatigue, and headache.*

Have you ever noticed that when you are talking with someone, you feel disengaged, agitated, tired, or even have a significant increase in fatigue and even pain symptoms? It's not uncommon for symptoms to present themselves during conversations, and then for those who experience symptoms to decide that social interactions trigger symptoms so are best avoided. This is like taking a sledgehammer to crack a walnut. When we unpick what is actually going on during these conversations we can see what can be altered.

As with everything Energy-flow, we are not going to blame Denise for off-loading and using Sandra. We are taking the perceptual position of empowerment and seeing how this can be an opportunity for Sandra to hone her skills of understanding what her true self is seeking to communicate.

When Denise offloads on Sandra she firmly remains in the "problem-space." The negative emotion that Denise felt during her experiences she re-experiences when talking to Sandra. Because she is not aiming to move out of the "problem-space" she stays stuck in the mud of the negative emotions triggered by her negative experiences. A harsher interpretation would be to say that Denise wallows in the negativity of her unpleasant experiences and almost enjoys moaning about how bad things are and how unfair her life is. There is no judgment of Denise, it is a simple observation that she has developed a habit of focusing on what is going wrong without taking any steps to put it right.

If you pause for a moment, I'm sure you can think of someone you know like this, someone who has that tendency to always want to talk about what is going wrong without really wanting to change anything. As you think about this person, you may already begin to feel your energy draining.

The solution is simple but not easy. When we get into a pattern of interacting with someone, making changes to our behavior pulls us out of our comfort zone because an energetic dynamic exists. Allowing yourself to step out of your comfort zone in order to allow your true self to flow will facilitate the reduction in symptoms. Let's look at what to do when faced with situations like this. One key way to prevent boredom and therefore increases in fatigue during conversations and social interactions is to remain *engaged* rather than *passive*. We have all had the experience of being passive where we slip into the background and disengage from what is taking place. This always triggers boredom, and fatigue ensues. A client was telling me recently that his girlfriend's sister had come for the weekend and on the Saturday when they were together he was feeling an increase in groggy fatigue. His thoughts went to the activities they might be doing and whether his symptoms would increase. He was focusing on his fear of symptoms and whether he was "overdoing it." This is one of the most common patterns of perception that can be extremely distracting. The idea of, "am I overdoing it?" creates fear because there is missing information and it leads us down a path away from why the symptoms are present in that moment. For my client his tendency was to disengage and become passive when his girlfriend's sister was around. Being passive is like tuning-out, taking a back seat, not involving yourself. Because being passive triggers boredom, fatigue symptoms quickly follow. The solution? To find some way of engaging in the social interaction, the conversation or to go and do something else.

When you are engaged rather than passive you are in a better position to affect the direction of the conversation. Changing the course of the conversation is a useful point—this could be through changing the subject. The final point with this example is if you are conversing with someone you are close with and can be honest with, you could invite them to move from the "problem space" into a "solution space." As a listener the energy is completely different when you are talking with someone who is relaying a problem and in doing so moving towards a solution, as compared with a person who is sitting in the problem space without any intention of moving. A way of saying this could be:

*"I hear what you are saying and I know that this is all really tough and it sounds pretty unpleasant. I'm thinking though that we need to be figuring out how to resolve this. I'm not sure it's great for you (and for me) to be going over this without the intention that we are going to find a solution or move towards a positive outcome."*

I would encourage you to find your own way of saying this; however, being clear of your intention will be beneficial for you and your relationships. The second trap is where we have a desire to help and in doing so we force ourselves into a position of having to offer advice and guidance. Usually this pressure is unconscious and is a little bit like a switch that is flicked on inside.

Here's an example of Pattern 2.

> *John was in his mid-fifties, and his daughter Susie was in her twenties. Every week Susie would come to visit her dad and talk about what had been going on in her life; minor problems with work and boyfriends. John suffered from chronic fatigue syndrome, anxiety, and panic attacks. Every week when Susie visited he would experience an increase in his symptoms when talking with her. John had an unconscious belief that in order for him to effectively support Susie, he had to offer advice, guidance, and solutions for her, whenever she faced problems and difficulties in her life. Each week an unconscious switch would flick, and he would place enormous pressure on himself to offer some advice and guidance. He believed it was his responsibility to solve Susie's problems, even though she wasn't asking for that level of input.*
>
> *When I started working with John, my first thought was that Suzie was burdening him as outlined in the pattern 1, above; however, he was adamant that this was not the case. Suzie didn't*

*have significant problems and it was certainly not her tendency to wallow or try to offload. What was evident as John spoke was his desire to support his daughter, and understandably so. But to John support meant offering advice and guidance; if he wasn't saying anything to her, he felt he wasn't really supporting her. To begin with we tried a little experiment; I instructed John to remain silent and just listen to Suzie next time she came, rather than his usual tactic of jumping in and trying to offer advice and guidance. I reassured him that simply providing a safe space for her to speak was sufficient support and, in fact, he didn't need to say anything in order to show support. He seemed happy enough to jump on board with our experiment and report back next session. When his next session arrived the results he reported were interesting. The first success was that he didn't experience an increase in symptoms during or after Suzie's visit. This was a major step forward. He did report, however, that he felt pretty frustrated with not being allowed to speak at all when she was discussing aspects of her life. He was aware of the urge to have to help and he recognized what almost felt like a compulsion to offer advice. This was the crucial piece. The next step was for John to be able to consciously trust his intuition and only offer advice to Suzie if he felt it bubbled up from his intuition, his true self rather than from compulsion. This was the middle ground we were looking for where he was ale to effectively switch off the compulsion to have to offer some sort of solution, advice or guidance.*

What I found particularly interesting was how pervasive and common it was to be driven by an urge to have to help or rescue people. I became aware that to some degree I was exhibiting this myself. I could see that as a natural helper and healer I would spring immediately to try and help people, often out of compulsion rather than because it felt intuitively right to do so. I applied the principles to my own life and was surprised at the difference. I allowed myself to go through the steps outlined below, and this became the model of teaching for my clients who were also prone to have that compulsion.

If this is a pattern for you, follow the steps below and play with this for a week or two.

1. The first step is to pause, breathe, and remind yourself that every experience every person has is perfectly okay. We often think that it's "bad" to have uncomfortable experiences or feel uncomfortable emotions and this is often what drives us to try and help others. It's as if we can't bear them not being happy, which is pretty ridiculous when you stop and think about it, but is one of the underpinning motivators for trying to always offer advice. A different perspective is recognizing that there may be value in all experiences, and allowing someone to have their experiences is a valid part of life.

2. Allow other people to have their emotional experiences and resist the compulsion to try and shift their emotional experience. Embrace the idea that there is nothing inherently wrong with emotional feelings of any sort, and it is part of our human experience to feel the full range of emotions. It is not your job to stand in the way of someone else's emotional experience.

3. Learn to turn off that switch that compels you to try and solve a problem or offer advice and guidance. Wait until you intuitively feel that you have advice or guidance to offer (this advice or guidance will be offered without an attachment to the outcome or a compulsion to shift the emotional state of the person you are talking to).

## Type 2: The Fixer and Problem Solver

The fixer is a person who is scanning life for opportunities to rescue others by fixing their problems or seeking to shift their emotional state from negative to positive. While there is great value in being of service and helping others, the tendency of the fixer is to neglect themselves and act from a foundation of compulsion to rectify and solve other people's problems. The fixer radiates the energy of the victim vortex and as a result tends to attract people who crave fixing, or those who have a tendency to take advantage.

There is a great quote by Martin Luther King Jr, that despite being used in a political context in reference to racial inequality in the United States, has great relevance and understanding of empowerment and energy.

*"And whenever men and women straighten their backs up, they are going somewhere, because a man can't ride your back unless it is bent."*

We can only be taken advantage of, treated unfairly or victimized if we reside within the victim-vortex. It is our responsibility to take charge of ourselves, the way we act, the way we think, and the way we speak. It would be easier for the fixer to blame those who take advantage, I know, I've been in that space. However, that approach keeps us locked in the vortex, and history will repeat itself. What if nothing can harm us unless we allow it? This is the foundation for the idea that there are no victims or villains. We can only be unfairly treated if we are allowing ourselves to reside in the victim-vortex. As soon as we take responsibility for ourselves our energy changes and we leave the vortex behind.

To step away from the compulsion of fixing we need to consciously make a choice based on our intuitive nudges. Deep down you will know when something feels right. Underneath the compulsive instinct or urge will reside a deeper feeling. This is your True Self. The communication is always there, we simply have to create the space and allow ourselves to be guided by it. Like with everything else, this is a not a technique as such; however, we can map out the process in a series of steps, which gives us a point of focus and something to practice.

1. When you are either asked to help or do a favor; or even if you notice the urge to jump in and offer your fixing "services" before being asked. Stop and breathe before you act compulsively to offer help, try to help or simply take over by helping.
2. Check inside yourself for what you really feel is appropriate and right for you. This is the deeper intuitive nudge that resides underneath the compulsion.
3. Do what feels right for you, rather than simply trying to help or rescue.
4. It may feel awkward at first because you are so used to your old patterns of fixing and rescuing. However, as you break the cycle of rescuing followed by feeling overwhelmed or symptomatic, you will build a new pattern that will soon feel right.
5. What is important to remember is that you are not helping yourself or the other person by rescuing them. You

run the risk of disempowering them and facilitating a dependency on you that will only hurt them and you in the long run.

## Being You: The License to Be Yourself

In a world where conformity is king, it can be difficult to stand aside and do what feels right for you. Most people want to be nice, they want to get along and fit in. However, these attempts to fit in, say and do the "right thing" can block the real you.

Being you, the full expression of you, is vitally important to ensure we steer clear of the victim-vortex. Compromises lead us back down that path and suck us back into habits and practices that lead to low mood at best and symptoms at worst. It can be difficult if the usual pattern is to want to keep the peace, not rock the boat or upset the apple cart, and think it is going to be easier or safer to go along with the wishes of others. Of course this can be difficult if your mind has decided that the conditioned version of you is who you really are, or if you don't know or are confused about how you feel. At this stage keep things simple, do what feels right for you, pay attention to how you feel and you'll soon begin to recognize when you are abandoning your true self in favor of fitting in.

Bear in mind, as mentioned previously, doing something new feels strange at first, e.g. saying "no" once in a while, when you always say "yes" will push you out of your comfort zone, but this discomfort will be transient, so persist with what you know to be right, deep in your core essence.

Think of this as owning a license to be yourself. You don't have to explain yourself to anyone, you don't have to fit in or be concerned what others think, this license allows you to be yourself, fully and totally. This is not an easy ask, especially if you are familiar with justifying, explaining or defending your words and actions. The idea that you don't have to justify, defend or explain is massive. If you were to stop and think about it for a moment and review the last couple of weeks, how many times have you felt a compulsion to justify your actions or words? Can you imagine what it would feel like if you never had to justify or defend yourself ever again? I'm not suggesting that this is the case, but I am inviting you to consider significantly reducing the frequency of self-justifications. There will be times when your intelligent body sends indignation and your true self guides you to make a stand and defend your feelings or actions. However, these instances are rare, especially when we compare them with the usual frequency with which people act from a compulsion to defend their feelings or actions. If you recognize this pattern in yourself, follow the principles we have discussed previously in moving away from compulsions.

## Attuning to Body Rhythm

When we are being ourselves and in our own flow, there is a natural rhythm that accompanies our energy, this is very different from the compulsive urge we have to fix problems. However, when our energy is focused in our mind and we tend to be out of touch with our natural body rhythm. With busy lifestyles it is easy to get stuck on a timeline and jump back and forth between past and future, spending very little time in the here and now. You will recognize this state when you have a busy mind that is creating future scenarios and going over old situations and circumstances.

I would always notice this as a feeling of a tight band around my forehead. It would start with a mild tingling and slowly get more pronounced and would feel like I was being pulled forward by a leash attached to my head. I would be doing one thing while thinking about 6 others things that needed to be done. The more we think about activities B, C, and D while performing activity A, the more we get stuck in the mind and the more we detach ourselves from our natural body rhythm. The result is a buildup of tension within the body because the tendency is for the mind to push us to go quicker or harder as we as we lose touch with our true self.

To give you some further clues, here are some examples of operating on "mind-rhythm" as opposed to "body-rhythm." If you would answer "yes" or even "possibly" to these questions the exercise below will be of great value to you.

Do you:

- Have an almost constant sense of urgency without knowing why?
- Do several things at once most of the time?
- Find that your mind is always racing?
- Feel guilty when you sit down and do nothing?

- Always think about the next thing to do?
- Feel angry at people who do things slowly?
- Drive quickly, usually faster than needed, with a tendency to feel impatient with other drivers?
- Harbor a general feeling of impatience and intolerance in relation to others?
- Find yourself having arguments with friends, family, or colleagues quite frequently?
- Find that you are frequently critical of others and yourself?
- Find that you are always looking for the next "kick" or "fix" with a sense of agitation about the now moment?

Here's the process for attuning to body-rhythm.

1. Step off the timeline by bringing your attention back to the here and now. Allow yourself to focus on the activity you are engaged in right now without thinking about the next few activities to come.
2. Allow yourself to observe your breathing and begin to feel your body's energy and natural rhythm.
3. As you continue to do what you are doing, let yourself move in alignment with your natural rhythmic flow.
4. Feel the harmony that exists between you and what you are doing. Have the activity be an extension of you rather that something you are forcing or pushing.
5. Practice this process frequently so you train yourself to be aligned and connected to this natural body rhythm in the moment. You will find that there is much more of a flow to everything you do when in this state, rather than the usual feelings of tension that comes from mind pushing and forcing.

## The Bigger Lessons of Life

Many years ago I was working with a client who had been experiencing life in the role of victim in her relationships. She had been involved with a number of abusive men and in each instance it was only when she was in the relationship and she was trying to deal with the abuse that she realized she was in an abusive relationship. It was as if her ability to detect these men and situations before they happened was absent. She was hit in a blind-spot, and out of nowhere she would "find" herself in the same situation again without having seen it coming.

As we worked together and realigned her with her true self, she began to develop her awareness of the feelings and intuitive nudges that were seeking to guide her in a more beneficial direction. Over a period of time she was able to put boundaries in place to stop and then prevent herself from being unfairly treated and she then developed effective "antennae" for detecting people and relationships that would serve her and treat her as she wanted to be treated, rather than in an abusive manner. I will always remember the final time we met and she reported that she was happy, symptom-free, and in a healthy relationship. Since working with me her awareness of herself, her motivations, and behavior had developed and on review she noticed something very interesting. When she had been in abusive relationships she had other friends who were also in unhealthy or abusive relationships. Since creating behavioral and energetic shifts in herself, which enabled her to move out of the victim-manipulator-rescuer vortex, she noticed that she no longer had any friends who were in abusive relationships. It seemed that when in victim vortex she "attracted" both abusers and other victims. Having shifted she no longer "attracted" either.

In another example, a client was telling me about a situation at work, where a new member of staff had been brought on board. This new staff member was particularly ambitious and, from the perspective of my client, was happy to walk over whoever was in the way to climb the "greasy pole" to career success. Having initially developed a good working relationship and trust with this new member of the team, my client then found himself being the one walked over. He told me that the new member of staff had lied about him and turned other members of the team against him. The end result was that she had been promoted above him and he had lost the confidence of other members of staff, including managers. He left his company and moved to a different part of the country to take up a different job in a different organization. To my amazement, he then proceeded to tell me the same story. He experienced the exact same turn of events—exactly the same, almost nothing was different. What was also amazing was that as he was telling me he wasn't aware himself. It was only as he finished the story that the realization dawned on him. How could this possibly be?

I then reflected on other clients and my own life and it hit me; none of us see these situations coming. It's as if there are bigger lessons in life that we need to learn from, and somehow these situations and people are drawn to us and we find ourselves facing the same types of situations and the same types of people over and over again until we realize the common denominator: us. As I opened my eyes to this phenomenon, it was becoming apparent that in many instances the intensity, severity, and frequency of these events was on the increase. I was having clients come into my office telling me about a situation that had occurred two weeks ago and then something similar but more intense happening yesterday. What was going on?

What if spiritual notions of life lessons are actually right? An academic perspective would suggest that certain personality types, traits, and characteristics determine behavior and therefore play a significant role in life outcomes. It's also the case that there are those who suggest that sufferers of CFS, fibro, and related conditions have similar personality types. However, my sense is that it goes beyond this, and I have seen people with significantly different "personalities" experience overlaps in "life lessons."

While I'm not going to suggest that life lessons are necessarily true or set in stone, I am going to invite you to entertain some ideas that might be helpful in regaining health and experiencing greater peace of mind. What if, somehow the experiences you face in life are somehow drawn towards you in order for you to experience and master your life lessons? As a human being your tendency will be to fixate on the specifics of a situation, the people involved, and the circumstances. But there will be something going on in the background. Everything is energy, and as receivers and transmitters of energy, we will be attracting the energy of situations. This means that when something takes place in your life there is a strong possibility that something else is going on. If you feel strong emotions and you "find" yourself in a situation that triggers strong emotions, or even symptoms, there is a good chance that your life lessons are being triggered.

Now I am aware that new agers will lean towards the notion that everything happens for a reason, and maybe it does. The problem that exists with that idea is that your interpretation of what an event "means" has every chance of being completely wrong. The number of times I've heard people say, well this happened so it's obviously a sign that I shouldn't be doing that. My immediate thought is that there are potentially tens if not hundreds of ways of interpreting what "this" actually means and it may not relate in any way to doing "that."

Where does that leave us, and how is this helpful? My belief is that the starting point is to be open to the notion that there are patterns to our experiences and these patterns relate to our energy and our life lessons. I am not going to attempt to categorize life lessons here because it is beyond the scope of this book. There is, however, value in looking beyond the specific content and context of our experience. For example, if you find that you have a boss who seems to manipulate you into doing extra work and you get caught up in the content and context of that work in that situation, you might miss the fact that there are other circumstances with other people whereby you are manipulated either blatantly or subtly. A fixation with the people involved and the specifics mean you miss the big picture. Focusing outside of yourself and blaming life, people, situations, God, all mean that you fail to see beyond the details and understand the bigger picture, and crucially by judging other people you will fail to implement whatever lessons are needed to be learnt.

History repeats itself, so if you do have a boss who manipulates you or treats you badly and you suppress your true feelings, allow it to happen, blame your boss for being a bad person, talk, think, act, and believe that you are a victim, you will never recognize that there is a lesson to be learnt. In order to master your life lessons you need to recognize that whatever emotions you feel are about you, the people involved to a certain extent are irrelevant because if it weren't those people it would be someone else. This is exactly why jumping into making major lifestyle changes, like leaving a job or relationship should not be the first response. You don't want remove yourself from a situation and then find yourself in another identical situation. You might also find that memories of previous circumstances seem to appear out of nowhere. As we discussed earlier, memories can serve as a reminder that whatever is happening now is connected to something similar in the past. The course of action is not to talk to a therapist about the past situation it is to identify how you need to change your interaction with the current situation in order to allow your true self to flow.

Let's do a little exercise; take a moment and imagine being in someone else's shoes observing you, or that you are a neutral observer looking in at your life. Then as this neutral observer, answer these questions to give an insight into some potential life lesson patterns that may prove useful in looking beyond circumstances.

When reviewing your life in recent years

1. Do you find that you resist external events, have a strong desire to hold onto the status quo, and struggle to deal with changes in life circumstances?

2. Do you find that you are treated unfairly or taken advantage of

3. Do you find that you have difficulties in trusting others, are you suspicious of others' motives, especially in relation to you

4. Deep down, how do you feel about yourself—empty? Content? Do you prefer to give rather than receive—in fact do you find it difficult to receive unless you can find a very good reason for you to receive something

5. Do you find you strive to be liked or accepted by others? Have you noticed that there have been times when things have gone wrong or that you've fallen out with people when all you were trying to do was be popular and be liked?

6. Do people think you're very easy going? So easy going that you always do what other people want? Do you always find yourself fitting in with friends and family to the extent that you can't even remember the last time to considered what you wanted because you were too busy going along with what others wanted?

7. Do you feel uncomfortable to say how you feel? Are you much more comfortable talking about facts, "realities" and absolutes? Do you find yourself going quiet when you are in a position and you're asked to say how you really feel deep down?

8. Do people sometimes think that what you say and what you don't always match? Do you find that if you are really honest that you say what people want to hear, or say the right thing for the circumstances? Do you sometimes get

confused about whether you really believe what you say, or whether what you say is really true?

9. Do you find yourself always looking outside of yourself for answers? Do you find it difficult to know where you end and others being—so you can be unsure whether an opinion is your or someone else's? Do you struggle to know

10. Do you find you are looking into the future at what to avoid? Do you think you are driven by fear, or trying to avoid fear? Do you fear being alone?

11. In truth, do you think you are equal to others, or do you often find that you think others are better than you in some way or other? Do you find yourself struggling to find ways in which you are worthy or "as good as"?

Without doubt there will be some of those areas that resonate as a strong "yes" and others a mild "yes" or even a "no." What is important is to recognize that it is possible and plausible that the patterns occurring in your life are part of a bigger picture. Your job in mastering your life lessons is to be you, experience yourself, and trust the wisdom that is your true self.

CHAPTER 11

# Human Needs and Tapping
## Your Creative Flow

H AVE YOU EVER WONDERED WHY YOU DO WHAT YOU DO?
Why you make the choices that you make from everyday
decisions like what you might eat in a restaurant to what motivates
you to get out of bed in the morning? Do you ever wonder about the
actions and decisions of others and what lies beneath them? What is
that drives people to jump out of aeroplanes, run marathons, bake
cupcakes or even commit crimes? We are all unique and we have
our own idiosyncratic tendencies, however, there are commonalities
with regard to the types of deeper drives and needs that motivate our
actions.

In the early part of the 20th century, the field of humanistic psychology began to gain momentum, with its developing interest and
focus on human potential and our innate desire to move towards
self-actualization. The concept of self actualisation refers to the deep
drive to realize and fulfill one's potentials and talents. In 1943 the
famous psychologist, Abraham Maslow submitted a paper to the
journal of Psychological Review entitled *A Theory Of Human Motivation.* Maslow suggested that there was certain needs that were
common to all people and that much of our external behavior and
decision making was driven by a desire to satisfy these unconscious
needs. His paper put forward the theory that humans are motivated
or driven to fulfil these needs in a specific order. In an attempt to
categorize and disseminate what these unconscious motivators were,
he created what he called his *Hierarchy of Needs;* as each lower level
is satisfied, the person moves to the next level; the theory being that

an unmet need or deficiency drives a person's actions. Maslow proposed five levels in the hierarchy; the first two levels are physiological needs and safety needs, described by Maslow as basic needs for food, warmth, shelter, safety, and security. When these needs are met a person will graduate to the next two levels, which cover psychological needs. Belongingness and love relate to the need for friendship, connection, and intimacy, and esteem needs describe the need to status, success, and prestige. Finally there is self-actualization, which is about reaching one's potential, self-fulfillment, and personal development. Maslow's work was fairly groundbreaking and spawned a huge amount of interest. In the 1970s, a further three levels were added; cognitive needs for intellectual curiosity and understanding, aesthetic needs describing a search for beauty and form. These sit underneath the self-actualization needs, the eighth and final being transcendence, which is really about giving back and helping others reach their potentials.

So, how does this relate to health and recovery? There are two important points; first, Maslow was interested in what can go right with people rather than what can go wrong. This notion is particularly relevant to us because even though we need to be aware of symptoms and remember that they are a tap on the shoulder, we don't want to fixate on the idea that "I'm broken and need fixing." You are not broken and you have everything you need already within you to experience health and vitality. Having chronic fatigue or pain, anxiety, or depression can leave you stuck in a cycle of fixating on symptoms while you cut out huge chunks of your life. Continually focusing on symptoms and how to recover can keep you locked in a cycle of symptoms. Our focus needs to be on reconnecting with the true self and moving towards experiencing purpose and meaning in life. This is why once you have decided on a path to walk I advocate spending the minimum time on "getting well" and the maximum time on experiencing life as best you can. The second point is that when you suffer from a chronic health condition you lose touch with yourself, your needs, and how to get out of the mire and overwhelm that accompanies everyday life. When you get lost in symptoms you need a roadmap to guide you back to you, to help you find your purposes, passions, and sense of meaning. The final two chapters will teach you how to discover your needs and begin to create a life that is aligned with who you are and who you can be.

## Making Your Commitment to Yourself

Before we get into understanding how to address and satisfy our human needs and tapping into our creative flow, there is a crucial first step. You have to really want to be here, now, living in this body, walking in these shoes. Let me be clear, not wanting to be here and actually wanting to kill yourself are two very different things. Not wanting to be here often manifests as being stuck in a rut, hating your life, feeling out of control, and wishing you could be transported somewhere else, or having a sense of treading water and going through the motions; existing rather than thriving. When you are in this space your energy becomes contorted, mangled, and depleted. I know, I've been there, I've experienced the words in my head, "I really don't want to be here now." If you haven't experienced that at one time or another I would be amazed. If you have and it's becoming all too familiar then it's time to do something about it.

Life can often seem overwhelming even when you don't have to deal with symptoms of fatigue, pain, anxiety, and depression. Let's face it life is pretty brutal at times, but the expectation is that you either toughen up and crack on with it, or you break down in some way or other. Between holding down a job or forging a career, raising a family, or just getting through each day, the journey of life seems fraught with difficulties and bumps in the road. As we look out into the world it can be difficult to know where to turn as we are over-loaded with information that bombards us from every angle.

When we are experiencing overwhelm for whatever reason, it is very easy to slip into the energetic space that we don't really want to be here. Life can seem too hard. When this happens we slide down the scale from being aligned with our true self to being misaligned, from high consciousness to low. Imagine yourself as a very power-ful source of energy, when you don't want to be here your energy becomes fractured and fragmented, it splinters off into a thousand different directions leaving you feeling drained. When this happens you'll find that nothing seems to go your way, you feel like you are going round in circles or walking through treacle. When your energy is splintered and shattered it's a bit like throwing a bouncy ball in a small room, it's unpredictable and destructive.

What I am going to ask you to do in this part will have a galva-nizing impact on your vibrancy. Your energy will begin to align in a cohesive formation, harmonizing like a channel of water flowing effortlessly downstream.

1. Make a decision that you really want to be on the planet. This could start with an intention, the statement that I want to be here. Really feel this in your body, this is not some trivial mental affirmation, this is a deep body-centered statement of intent that needs to resonate with your core in order to align you with your true self. Be curious about how this feels. You may notice resistance or fear, especially if you are in a space of overwhelm, confusion, low energy or pain. If you find this difficult, I would suggest revisiting this idea every day for the next week and each time notice how you feel. There is no right and wrong way to feel with this, it is simply part of the alignment process.

2. Once you have set your intention, and made your decision that you want to be here, the next step is to back up that decision with a reason for being here. I would recommend something general like, fulfilling your potential, having as much fun as possible, really engaging in things you really love, etc. The reason has to be for you, it can't be for someone else. Deciding you want to be here for your children or to cook for your partner are not reasons that honor and validate you. Your decision needs to be for you. As with step 1, you might want to feel into this for a few minutes every day for a week and notice how it feels in your body. You can hone your reason or reasons using your intuitive feelings as your guide.

## Going Beyond Survival Mode

Even when you have made your commitment to yourself, the pace of modern life combined with chronic symptoms can leave you feeling detached from life and yourself. It is not uncommon to feel like you are watching life from inside a bubble, unable to fully take part. It can seem like you can barely muster the energy to get through the day. This is the survival mode of life and can feel like a trap you've fallen into and can't climb out; like being stuck in a trance, going through the motions without really being present or engaged in life. It can creep up on you just like a rut, and until to stop and look at your life you probably won't detect you're in survival mode. Vibrationally it is heavy and dense and pulls us away from our high-consciousness connection with true self.

Even though you are rarely present with open awareness when in survival mode, it is different from daydreaming, which is a natural part of life. Being present in as many moments in life as possible has value, however, there is an ebb and flow about presence, sometimes it will flow with effortless ease and other times it will be unnatural. We never want to force ourselves to be present. Gently inviting ourselves to align by bringing attention back into the body without force or getting into the mind is the key. If you find yourself day-dreaming let it flow, recognize that it is different from feeling chronically disengaged where you might feel you are running on autopilot. The risk in today's environment is to give yourself a hard time because you think you should be mindful and present in every moment. This route usually ends up with getting stuck in the mind and drifting down the consciousness spectrum. Practice open awareness and let yourself flow, avoid beating yourself or setting standards, stipulations, and expectations for yourself. We want to nudge ourselves back to self-healing not baseball bat ourselves over the head. Our route away from survival mode is to begin to engage in life, to embrace life, and be a little more conscious about what we are doing and how it feels.

Maybe you could entertain this idea: have your intention be that you are going to get the most out of everything you do, you are going to have as much fun and enjoyment as you possibly can. The way we approach things has an enormous impact on both the way we feel as we do something, and the outcomes of what we are doing. There is a caveat here, it is important for us to understand that there is a natural up and down to life, some days we will feel happier and more upbeat than others and we simply have to accept that. Everything in life goes around in cycles, from the seasons to our moods, being "on" and happy is simply not realistic. We have periods of expansion and periods of contraction; times of growth and times of contemplation and reflection. These occur naturally and cannot be forced. So as with every aspect of Energy-flow, we align with deeper feelings.

Engaging with life in every moment does not mean forcing oneself to be happy and gregarious in every moment, it means being present and conscious, practicing open awareness.

There is tremendous pressure to "be on your game" and feel great at all times in today's culture. Status is more than the car you drive, the career, the houses or gadgets, status comes with experiences and performance. In today's society we have to achieve, have varied life experiences, which we rank on a bucket list, and be "out there" and happy. Flaunting our amazing life experiences on Facebook, Instagram, and Twitter has become mandatory as we seek to promote the perception of success, achievement, and happiness. The irony is that time spent on social media seems to add to levels of unhappiness, which probably arises from the perceptions of others' successes coupled with a disconnection from real life. It is at these times when our tendency to compare ourselves to others really comes to the fore. Comparison is an exercise that we invite children to begin doing at a young age and in some instances it can facilitate high achievement and in many others it can be the catalyst for self-flagellation and excessive negativity. If you are remotely prone to episodes of depression you will know all about comparison. When emotion builds up in the stress bucket the self-evaluation valve goes off in the brain and the downward spiral of self-flagellation begins. The solution is the same. Attune to feelings, align with true self; thinking will make you feel worse and take you down the consciousness spectrum.

## Attaining Clarity of Motivation and Intention

As we take steps to engage more fully in life the next step is to be clear about our intentions, purposes, and motivations. We need to know why we are doing what we are doing. Far too often we go about our daily lives without really making conscious decisions about what, why, how, and when we do what we do. It is very easy to drift along in a semi-conscious trance-like state, mindlessly moving from one activity to the next. We've all had that experience of wondering where the day went as we get lost in the "same old, same old."

Much of our behavior is unconscious, so we tend to replicate the same patterns over and over. The result being that we rarely make a conscious decision in the moment; instead we rely on what we've

always done in the way we've always done it. Running on autopilot to
a degree is an integral part of being human; we learn things quickly
and consign them to the unconscious, so we can focus our conscious
attention on something else. The problem arises when we allow ourselves to be completely governed by our past conditioning and our
unconscious dictates every decision we make whether it is right for
us in this moment or not. However, just as in the previous section I
was not suggesting that we need to force ourselves to be present and
mindful in every moment, so I am not suggesting that we have to
be present and making every decision a conscious decision. Making
decisions takes energy, so making a huge number of decisions can
feel draining. This is why there is great value in automating certain
aspects of life. Highly successful people tend to implement certain
routines either for specific activities or at certain times of the day.
Examples can include having a certain morning routine or ritual, or
having a set routine at the gym rather than making a series of decisions about each little thing that you do.

However, while there is value in automating certain activities and
times of the day, these routines need to be consciously constructed
at the outset based on an idea or notion of what will be or is already
effective. So if you have an automated morning ritual of getting up,
preparing coffee, spending fifteen minutes doing yoga, then reading
for 15 minutes before showering, that needs to be based on some evidence that implementing this routine facilities good "performance"
for you throughout the day. What is also important is that you
implement open awareness to ensure you are still feeling and conscious while going through your practice. This type of consciously
created routine or ritual is very different from an unconscious rut.
Too frequently we create habits and practices unconsciously, meaning that we find ourselves just doing the same things over and over
without having made a choice in the first instance. Or we get caught
in a rut because we thought we were choosing a certain path that
served us at one point in time, but now we're bored with it, yet we
haven't made a change. So a consciously created productive ritual
that supports health and performance is valuable while an unconscious rut that we drift into is likely to negatively impact our health
and performance.

Therefore our decision-making practices are an incredibly important part of life. Too few decisions and you are drifting through life

in unconscious mode playing out your unconscious programming and conditioning, and too many decisions and you'll feel drained and agitated. Our aim is to allow ourselves to feel guided by our true self. You will have experienced this in your life; a time when you something just felt like the right decision and it didn't seem to require any effort, it seemed to flow through you. This is what we want to encourage and develop.

Through the practice of open awareness you can be aware of how your body feels and this means you can detect emotional and intuitive feedback. We can feel energy as it moves through our body and make decisions for us that are right for us in this moment. When I was younger and went through a period of anxiety and overwhelm, it got to the point that my head was so cluttered and messy that I had no choice but to get out of the way and let go. Something took over me and I had a sense of an energy flowing through me guiding me. It was almost like being sat on a horse where all I can do was observe the route the horse took; because I knew I couldn't control the horse I don't bother trying, I imagined sitting back and observing with curiosity. The horse was of course my true self, flowing like an energy. Another metaphor that was familiar for me was having the sense that a cord of energy, almost like a cylinder of water extended out of my chest and pulled me along. All my thinking brain needed to do was observe where I was being pulled. This cord of energy was my intuition and inner knowing, my navigational system.

If you would like to try this for yourself, start with the intention that you are going to be guided by your true self and create your own Energy-flow. Pick a day or maybe two and decide that you are going to be curious about where you "feel pulled," then effectively sit back and observe where your body pulls you. You will notice that your chattering mind will want to intervene and tell you what to do; however, all you need do is remind yourself that you are playing a little game for a few days and you are going to be guided. You might be surprised that your head will want to take you in one direction and your intelligent body might pull you in another. Go with your flow and notice how it feels.

When we allow ourselves to be pulled along or guided by our true self rather than the overbearing dictator that is the chattering mind, our motivation and drive serve our highest and best interests, and the outcomes are favorable.

## Developing Motivation

Where does motivation fit with allowing yourself to be guided? Is it that simple that we can metaphorically sit back and let our true self take the reigns while our chattering mind is given the role of interested observer? Do we need motivation to get going? Do you ever have the experience that you don't get things one because you don't have the motivation to get going? Or maybe you feel angry because you want to have motivation but you feel washed out and you don't really know where to start? Many people think motivation is something fixed, you either have it or you don't, it's either there or it's not. When it's not there frustrations can arise because it can be easy to fixate on the void that seems to be left where motivation *should* be. When we are aligned there is an Energy-flow through us and life can seem almost effortless. Hard work becomes passionate working, a slog becomes an essential experience en route to expressing who you are. When we are able to experience our Energy-flow, motivation is not a topic we necessarily consider because if an activity doesn't feel right we wouldn't do it. We would let go of any forcing and allow ourselves to be guided towards something that does feel right. In saying that, there are always going to be tasks, activities, and chores that need doing. You might feel drawn to read a chapter of that exciting new book, but your daughter needs to be driven to her cheerleading session, so that takes precedence. But when we are aligned a natural balance occurs, when you are not in alignment you will find that you are doing far too many things that you probably don't want to do. This is when motivation seems like a problem, which is ironic because this is when you really think you need motivation because you can't seem to get going. The most common solution to this problem is to resort to mental tactics or techniques to motivate yourself. While "talking yourself into the mood" and other such mental techniques may seem to work in the short term, they tend to keep you locked in the chattering brain and disconnected from your true self and Energy-flow. In the long term your motivation drops even lower and you could find yourself in a loop of trying different mind-centered motivational techniques. Willpower is the same, it's like a muscle that fatigues. This is one of the reasons why most New Year's Resolutions have amounted to an epic fail by early February. Willpower is called upon as the motivator because the mind has been the dictator. The true self in most instances isn't even consulted when these decisions are made.

In an ideal world we do want to be aligning with our true self and letting it take the reigns; however, motivation is tied up with how we feel physically. It's impossible to separate our energy levels, symptoms, mental clarity, and our desire or drive to get going. So when you are feeling sluggish or beset with symptoms or fatigue, how do you get going? Motivation, like emotion is fluid. For example, if there is a part of you that would like to start going to a regular yoga class but every time the day arrives you can't find the motivation to get yourself to the class, there are two things you need to bear in mind. First, was your initial decision to take up yoga based on aligning with your true self or were you thinking that you should take up yoga because you've read countless articles online espousing the health benefits of yoga, so you really should? If it is the latter, I would encourage you to park the idea of the yoga class for the time being. There may come a point in the future when you recognize that your motivation is intrinsic and comes from inside you. If and when that happens then you'll find it easier to get to the class. Second, your motivation will develop. If you have decided that you really want to experience that yoga class you might need to give yourself a push to begin with, but remind yourself that your motivation is fluid and will develop. Motivation is not fixed or set in stone. Many people fear that if their motivation levels are not currently present they never will be. That simply isn't the case. Motivation is influenced in numerous ways, so giving yourself that push today will help develop and foster motivation for tomorrow.

When you look at your current life and the activities that you are involved in, what activities do you do because you are being guided from within, and how many are you doing because of external influences? External influences are called extrinsic motivators in the field of psychology and they refer to any external reward ranging from others people's feedback to achievements. While we are never going to remove the influence of external factors, focusing on them as the primary source for our motivation usually results in unsustainable efforts. If you find that it is difficult to get going, or that you never follow through there is a good chance that you are calling on extrinsic motivators to see you through. I'd like to invite you to redress the balance, develop your ability to be self-motivated by feeling where you are drawn, where you feel pulled by your true self.

## Meeting Human Needs

Now we've covered making your commitment to yourself and some simple elements of motivation, let's get back to understanding our human needs and how to satisfy them in order to improve our health and life experience. Abraham Maslow's work on human needs offers the definitive academic perspective and guide to human needs; however, there are many variations on the theme of meeting human needs. Our focus is on addressing needs that will facilitate optimum health, which in turn is linked with happiness and peace of mind.

Take a look at the list below and review which of these needs are satisfied in your life and which are not. When you are in alignment with your true self you will naturally move towards fulfilling these needs. However, the more out of alignment you become the greater the chance that fewer of these needs will be met. This list is not meant to be prescriptive, rather allow it to be your guide, identify where there are gaps and where you could make changes.

1. INTERACTIONS AND CONNECTIONS WITH PEOPLE. There are two parts to this need; the first is feeling part of a community, be that a family system or part of a wider group. The second part is experiencing one-to-one connections. From both an evolutionary and a metaphysical perspective we are connected to each other, and the absence of connection triggers loneliness and stress. Evolutionary psychology would suggest that we evolved in nomadic tribes living in close proximity to each other. We lived and died with a common purpose and a deep sense of connection with our "tribe." This is something that is absent in today's society. We live in homes and apartments with no common sense of purpose or connection. When a society is in crisis it tends to pull together and in the absence of connection and common purpose we see increases in crime and antisocial or dysfunctional behavior as well as increases in chronic health problems. Following the 9/11 attacks in New York, there was a great sense of connection and common purpose that arose out of those tragic events. The interesting outcome was a drop in crime rates and war veterans reporting fewer experiences and symptoms of PTSD. I have witnessed this

phenomenon on a small scale with clients who have experienced significant shifts when other family members are in crisis. There is something tribal that is hardwired and drives us to connect with and help each other. The metaphysical or spiritual view would be that we are all one, we are "waves on an ocean," all part of a single consciousness experiencing itself in an infinite number of ways.

2. CREATIVE EXPRESSION AND CREATIVITY. What are creativity and creative expression? Traditionally we tend to think of being creative as exclusive to pursuits in art or music; however, creativity is a wider concept that represents an expression of you in any field or endeavor. You could be creativity expressing yourself coding a computer program or running on the football field. Creativity in any area of life represents a connection to our true self, when we are aligned creativity will flow in the form of insight and wisdom. When we are not in alignment we tend to over think and get cluttered in the mind.

I'm not going to try and teach you how to be creative here; there are many resources available in books and online. What I will say is that whether you think of yourself as creative or not, creative energy is a part of your Energy-flow. Whenever you have been playful, outrageous, absurd, off-the-wall, or spontaneous, you have been allowing your creative energy to flow. Stifling it arises through shutting down those aspects of yourself and living within your mind. The simplest way to open up to your crave flow is to allow yourself to be guided as we talked about in the last section. Be playful, be spontaneous, breathe, connect with your body, and give yourself time to engage in activities that allow you to be a little more creative.

If you were to take a moment and review your life, are you allowing your creative energy to flow, are you engaging in activities that facilitate an unfolding of your true self, or are you shut-down, and engaged in activities that are monotonous and require nothing in the form of creative expression? I commonly ask clients about creativity and frequently they tell me about creative outlets they had in the past, activities they engaged in, but for some reason these don't form a part of their lives anymore. As we get older, our lives become narrower, we tend to define ourselves quite tightly, and as we leave old pastimes and pursuits behind, we rarely replace them with new ones. This is when we get stuck in ruts and creative expression eludes us. This situation gets amped up considerably when you suffer from a chronic health condition and entire chunks of your life are lanced in an attempt to save energy. The solution is knowing the importance of creative expression, through alignment with your true self and through activities that facilitate your Energy-flow.

A useful exercise is to review what activities you have done in the past and feel into whether they are activities you would like to bring back into your life. Remember, this is not a thinking exercise it is a feeling exercise. If you decide that there are not activities from the past you would like to be doing now, I would suggest reviewing anything that you've always wanted to do but never had the chance, as well as looking at what other people do. Even if you pick one new activity or pastime; take the steps towards bringing that into your life. What can you do today, what's the first step you need to take?

The primary block to creativity is the perceived burden of life chores and maintenance tasks, all the things we have to do and have to be done in a certain way or at a certain time. It's very easy for life to consist almost entirely of work and household chores and our lives to become narrower and narrower.

Here's a little fun exercise you could play with.

PART ONE:
1. Make a list of all the activities that fill your life, including work, household chores.
2. Think about the amount of time you spend on each activity and give a percentage score—for example: work 65 percent; household chores 10 percent; playing tennis with friends, 1 percent, and so on.
3. As you look at the list and the scores what do you feel?
4. Take a different color pen and review and change your percentages to ones you would prefer (for example: household chores, 7 percent; tennis with friends, 5 percent; and so on.)
5. Are you prepared to make changes so you can attain these new percentages?

PART 2: KEEPING LIFE FRESH, INTRODUCING NEW ACTIVITIES
1. Get your pen and paper at the ready.
2. Sit back and spend a minute or two breathing and connecting with yourself.

3. With pen in hand, write a list of all potential creative, fulfilling, fun, and purposeful activities that pop into your consciousness or awareness. Avoid letting your head or analytical left-brain get in the way, simply let the ideas flow out of your pen, as if the pen is an extension of your own inner consciousness.

4. When you've finished, think back over your life and write down activities that you have done in the past that have been expressions of your creativity or activities you have really enjoyed, whatever they may be.

5. Finally think about things you've always wanted to do but have never done, or even activities that other people engage in or practice.

6. Once you have your list go back through it and feel which of the items are the most important.

7. What additional resources would you need to be able to begin these activities now?

8. What obstacles are standing in your way—what would stop you from doing these activities?

9. Do you need a series of steps to build up, and if so what can you begin doing today?

3. SENSE OF PURPOSE AND MEANING. I often encounter the idea that we need to identify our life's purpose in order to be fully happy, and possibly fully healthy. I disagree with this idea. I don't believe we necessarily have a single life purpose. My experience is that believing that you need to find your purpose only leads to additional internal pressure, which contributes to health problems and unhappiness. Also, purpose and meaning don't have to be solely future focused. Again, there can be a pressure with having to achieve when we are constantly focused on purpose as tied with future goals. I'm not saying there is anything wrong with goals as such, however, I do feel that having a sense of direction can be a little more empowering and less pressured than having life goals.

I would encourage you to embrace the idea of life purposes rather than seeking a single purpose. I'm not suggesting that you shouldn't have a single life purpose if you already have one, I am just suggesting you embrace multiple purposes if you don't. Make conscious decisions about what you choose to do and not to do. If you look at your life and see that you are engaged in a stack of activities that do not serve your sense of meaning and purpose, consider removing them from your life. Don't do things because it's what you've always done or because you think you should. You are here to experience yourself as fully as you possibly can, so seek out those things that help you do that.

Meaning and purpose can be light and fun as well as serious and heavy. You can derive a sense of meaning and purpose from goofing around with a friend as well as when volunteering for a local charity or engaging in spiritual practice. In fact seeking out a wide variety of experiences and activities helps to fully experience the different aspects of who you are.

4. SENSE OF AUTONOMY OR CONTROL OVER YOUR DIRECTION—PERSONAL FREEDOM. What you are going to find is that the starting point for addressing many of your human needs comes through aligning with your true self. A statement I have heard numerous clients make over the years is that "I am not in control of my life" or "my life is not my own." When we allow ourselves to be sucked into an external flow we lose our sense of self.

Do you feel that you are directing your own life? If yes, great. If not, what would need to change in order for you to begin to feel that you are taking the reins and you are not a pawn in life's uncertain game of chance? Suffering from chronic symptoms can trick you into thinking that you are a victim of circumstance where you abandon any sense of autonomy. Addressing this starts with making decisions about what you do every day that are rooted in moving towards what feels right for you.

5. PHYSICAL ACTIVITY. Put simply we need to move, if you are not moving your body in one form or another your energy will be stagnant and this will exacerbate a variety of symptoms. What is important, however, is that you chose an activity that you enjoy. Exercising because you think you should is counter productive.

In my work with sufferers of CFS, I constantly invite my clients to see that it is not simply exertion that causes or triggers symptoms. When we put on our emotional glasses and view the world in this way, we can see that our intelligent body is responding to everything we are doing. There are two stories I would like to share about exercise and exertion.

*The first is a client, Sam, who was in her early thirties when she started working with me. She had CFS and was just able to function so that she could work part time. However, on the days she worked she would come home exhausted, attributing this to exertion. One session Sam told me that there was a birthday party for one of the girls, Julie, at the office and the plan was to head to a night club and go dancing. Sam had loved dancing before her CFS, but since her diagnosis and symptom increase she had completely curtailed her nightclub outings. However, as Julie was a good friend at work she really wanted to be there. Sam got home from work, exhausted as usual and was deeply concerned that she'd either never be able to make it out or worse, if she did make it to the club she was worried that she'd never make it home. She called Julie thinking about pulling out but Julie smoothly talked Sam round and the decision was final. Sam dragged her heavy body upstairs and got changed. Was she making a massive mistake, how was the night going to pan out? She took a taxi to meet Julie and the rest of the girls and the night began. The group wasn't a big one and they were all good friends. They laughed, joked, and told stories and before long, Sam's symptoms were beginning to recede a little. When they got to the nightclub Sam's focus was on having a good time, she wasn't thinking about her symptoms or the potential ramifications of her night out; she was getting lost in the fun and going with her flow.*

*Sam and Julie danced until the early hours of the morning, both of them tired and exhilarated after the best night they'd had in years. Sam arrived home tired but not "symptom tired." She went to bed and went straight to sleep. When Sam awoke in the morning she got up as usual and got ready for work, then it hit her, there was no drastic increase in symptoms. How could this be? The symptoms she had experienced after work had dissolved when she went out and despite dancing all night her symptoms did not increase in fact they had all but disappeared What did this mean? Well, it proved to her that physical activity in and of itself did not cause physical symptoms, in fact quite the opposite. She had gone out feeling fatigue symptoms and as she started to enjoy herself, let go, and get into her Energy-flow her symptoms dissolved.*

The second story is the total opposite. This was the first client who came to me with CFS and told me that I was the only "alternative" therapist he had seen outside of mainstream.

*Dan was a guy in his mid-fifties and had been a personal trainer of sorts for the majority of his working life. Exercise was his life, yet he told me that exercise caused symptoms. He loved exercise, so he said, so if what I was saying was right how on earth did it cause symptoms. He gave me example after example of times when he as exercising and his symptoms increased. This didn't make sense to me, if he truly loved what he was doing and his intelligent body was feeding that back with high vibrational emotions. I was asking him questions trying to find the hidden low vibrational emotions that might be contributing to his symptoms increases, but nothing was forthcoming. Then at session four he told me that an old injury had been playing up in recent months, which precluded him from doing all the sport he loved and all he could do was swim and walk, and he didn't like swimming or walking.*

*"So you don't actually enjoy the exercise you're doing?"*

*"Well, actually no, I really don't enjoy this exercise."*

*"Why are you exercising then?"*

*"Because I have to, I have high blood pressure and cholesterol, and it's who I am."*

*"Let me see if I have this right, you are exercising on a daily basis at the moment because you think you have to, not because you actually enjoy it? I appreciate you've been involved in exercise all your life and it's part of who you are, but right now, you really are not enjoying it?"*

*"No, I guess I'm not. Are you telling me that I don't have to exercise?"*

*"Yes, that's exactly what I'm telling you. Forcing yourself to exercise when you don't want to is triggering frustration and agitation, which is leading to an increase in your symptoms. It's not simply that exercise causes symptoms, it's the feedback your intelligent body is sending about the exercise."*

*This was a revelation for Dan, and a difficult one for him to take on board. His sense of identity was wrapped up with being a person who exercised daily and loved it. He was now faced with being a person who didn't love all exercise, in fact he really didn't want to exercise at the moment, and the forcing himself was impacting his CFS symptoms.*

What we can learn from this is that if you are going to exercise be guided towards it. Exercise because it feels right and you enjoy it, pick something that you do enjoy. Exercising because you think you should will more than likely lead to more symptoms.

6. TRANSPERSONAL CONNECTION. When it comes down to it, most people have a sense of something greater than themselves. Be this a religious or spiritual faith or feeling or just a sense of unity and connection with all that is. If this does not feature in your life it is unlikely to be significant in your journey back to health. However, it can help if you can see a bigger picture and join the dots, as it does to understand experiences as life lessons where we can remove judgment and flow with greater ease. The important piece in getting well is finding yourself, if you discover a connection with everything else along the way embrace it.

## Finding Your Passions and Purposes

We're going to end this chapter with a couple of exercises that you may find useful.

In our modern brain-centered culture, it is so easy to buy into the mass consciousness ideas of what you should like, what you should do, and how you should feel about things. This is a trap, a trap that separates us from ourselves. Your job as a human being is to experience who you are and to live the full expression of yourself. Even though it may currently feel as if there is nothing that ignites your passion, those passions and purposes are simply lying dormant inside, waiting to be tapped, to be activated. Our job in this process is to help you reconnect with your true self in order to realize the potentials that lie within you, and to spend more time in a higher consciousness state of passion and joy.

There are many people who feel they have an absolute purpose for being on the planet and they strive diligently to find that purpose. I am of a different mindset. I believe we have the opportunity to develop fresh purposes as we live to acquire experience and live to our potential. What does this mean? Because of the natural tendency to strive, to force and push in order to attain, when this is applied to the notion of purpose the result is usually discomfort and a feeling of emptiness and unworthiness. By stepping into a space of not knowing and curiosity we can allow ourselves to be guided without force, trusting our intuitive core feelings as our true self offers hints and nudges us as we move along our path.

We all have the potential to develop many multilayered purposes and passions, however, they have to flow without judgment, restriction, or limitation. Simply allow yourself to follow what excites you. Let it be simple, avoid overwhelming yourself. All experience is valuable experience and you will be guided to where you need to be regardless of your chattering mind.

If you are feeling playful, you might want to try this. If it feels too familiar with the exercise in the previous section then leave it, or come back to it later.

1. Get a pen and a blank sheet of paper.
2. Draw a small circle in the center of the sheet and write "Happiness" in the circle.
3. Then, think about the times in your life when you have been happy. When were you happy and what were you doing?
4. Write these as words or phrases outside your central circle.
5. Draw circles around what you have written and connect them to the central circle.
6. Do your entries have anything in common?
7. How many of these items that make you happy are in your life now?
8. Take a new sheet of paper and write "Purpose" in a circle in the center
9. Write down when you have felt a real sense of purpose— what you were doing and who you were with. Take your time with this, and go back in time as far as you like.
10. Are there things that you know would give you a sense of purpose and meaning but are not in your life? Write these down.
11. Look back over both sheets of paper—have you missed

anything that would ignite your passion? Are there any new things that you would like in your life but for whatever reasons are not currently in your life? Write them down.

12. Decide for yourself which of these are most important and think about when you might want to start getting these happiness and sense of purpose-provoking activities in your life.

13. Are there additional resources you would need to be able to get these things in your life or begin these activities now?

14. What obstacles are standing in your way—what would stop you from moving forward and getting these things in (or back in) your life?

15. Do you need a series of steps to build up, and if so, what can you begin doing today?

16. Stick your pieces of paper next to your computer so that you see them every day.

17. Notice how you feel when you look at your entries.

When to do the exercise:

Make a commitment that you are going to work through your list, and start including some of your new activities this week. As best you can, use this list, update it from time to time, and keep bringing those new things in your life to facilitate your ongoing journey towards health and happiness with passion and purpose.

# CHAPTER 12

# Life Design and Creation

I MAGINE FOR A MOMENT A SCENE IN A SCIENCE FICTION MOVIE where the main character is the captain and lead scientist on mission into space to save planet earth. He's sitting in a dark room hunched over a table scribbling something on a large piece of paper, struggling to take in what he has just encountered. As their ship was traveling through space in search of solutions to the crises faced by planet earth, they encountered what they thought were aliens from another planet. The aliens turned out to be inhabitants of earth who had traveled back in time 100,000 years to deliver a message. The message they delivered was that the answers to the problems faced by planet earth were not going to be found out in space, they were on earth. Now the team had to return without the magical extra terrestrial solution they thought they needed, rather all they had is this knowledge that somehow they would need to disseminate and deliver.

Earth's future inhabitants told the captain that even though the crises on earth seem beyond all control, humans are magnificent creators, and everything that exists in their reality is part of their own creation, both individually and collectively. Human beings are connected to an infinite intelligence and consciousness, and it is from this consciousness that all life emerges. As a scientist, this was very difficult for the captain to take in. He, like his crew of scientists, believed that humans were nothing more than robotic pawns controlled by conditioning and genetics, living their lives in a directionless, purposeless universe.

As he sat scribbling on his paper he reviewed many aspects of his life and the lives of those he loved. He was beginning to see that the news he had been given made perfect sense. He could see how life on earth could be different, better. He could see the extent to which humanity felt enslaved, and while they thought of themselves as victims of circumstances beyond their control, they were actually only a few steps away from directing and gaining mastery over life. He had been given the keys to mastery, to unlock the gateway to changing the lives of everyone on earth by giving them this new knowledge: the knowledge to redesign and create lives filled with purpose and passion rather than lives of strife and crises.

How would you feel if you sat in the movie theatre watching this movie, and then found yourself transported into the movie and into the body of the captain? How would it feel to know that life may not be as you had thought, that you may be radically different from your current conception of yourself, and that you have a far greater influence over your reality and experience than you had once thought? Would that frighten you, excite you, both?

As we move through this final chapter, we are going to unearth some of the ideas that you will need to redesign your life and move forward as the creator of your own experience and reality. You may be familiar with the type of material you will be reading here or it may be completely new to you. Either way if you allow yourself to integrate this material it will give you an entirely different perspective of your life, your health, and the world around you.

## Attraction and Conscious Creation

Have you ever had the experience of waking up and thinking or feeling that this is going to be a bad day; then you bang your head as you step in the shower, overfill the coffee pot, somehow leave late for work and then get stuck in unexpected traffic? Or maybe you have had the feeling that a colleague doesn't like you and the more you think about it the more obvious it seems that they don't like you. Are you psychic or are you somehow creating this, and how would you know the difference?

You are probably familiar with the notion of a "self-fulfilling prophesy," where what you expect to happen just seems to happen. This is most certainly the case when other people are involved. In psychology this has been called The Pygmalion Effect and was most effectively demonstrated by psychologist Robert Rosenthal and school principal Lenore Jacobson. In their experiment, school teachers were informed that on the basis of some psychological tests, certain students were expected to improve significantly during the year, despite having no shown any particular academic prowess up to that point. The teachers unknowingly began acting differently towards those students because they were expecting them to begin to shine as the year progressed. The students in turn unknowingly shifted their own beliefs and expectations about themselves and performed significantly better on intelligence based assessments than the other students. The teachers did not know that the children had been randomly selected and had not been given a special test, and the students did not know that the teachers had been given additional information about their expected improvements in performance.

Given this remarkable yet not surprising result, you would probably expect the reverse to be true, and you would be right. American teacher, researcher, and activist Jane Elliot conducted a study where the students in her class were separated according to eye colour—a blue-eyed group and a brown-eyed group. She told those in the blue-eyed group that they were superior and cleverer and that brown-eyed people were slower, poorer listeners, and not as smart. The brown-eyed group were made to wear a collar to identify them, they were not allowed to drink from the water cooler or play with the blue-eyed group. Whereas the blue-eyed group were given extra privileges, allowed additional time at breaks, and sat at the front of the class while the brown eyed group sat at the back.

The impact on both groups was significant. Attitudinally the blue-eyed group became more arrogant and bossy and even engaged in bullying members of the brown-eyed group. In contrast the brown-eyed group became more withdrawn, dejected, and disenfranchised. There was also an impact on performance with the blue-eyed group showing improvements in academic tests and the brown-eyed group showed a dip in academic performance. On the second day of the experiment, Elliot changed the groups and the effects reversed, though they were not as intense.

What is evident with the Pygmalion Effect is something of a circular pattern where our beliefs and expectations affect our actions and behavior in relation to others; this in turn affects others' beliefs and expectations, which impacts their actions and behaviors.

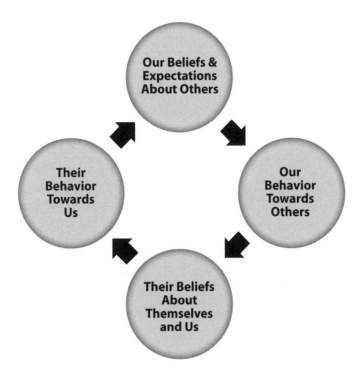

When I worked as a psychologist in research and management consulting, I managed a project that sought to help reduce the number of accidents in the workplace for young people on government training programs in heavy industry. As you might expect, the research program involved gathering data from a broad range of organisations including those where there were a high number of accidents, as well as those at other end of the spectrum where there were no accidents. The research findings exemplified the Pygmalion Effect in action. In organisations where young people were treated as children, given odd jobs like sweeping floors or clearing rubbish, poorly trained, not trusted with responsibility, and isolated from teams, the number of accidents were high. Conversely, where young people were treated as equal members of the team, trusted and given responsible jobs, and effectively trained, they responded and performed effectively, didn't play-up, mess around, get into mischief, or cause accidents.

While the Pygmalion Effect gives an insight into the notion of a self-fulfilling prophecy when other people are involved, we still need to explore those instances where other people are not involved yet things seem to either go right or wrong for us. Is this just luck or coincidence?

If you remember in Chapter 4, we talked about the spectrum of high and low vibrational consciousness.

As we align with our true selves we move into higher vibrational consciousness with the off-shoot that life seems to flow and we experience less suffering. But how can we impact what shows-up in our experience of life? Are we really creating our own reality? There has been something of a surge of interest in the "law of attraction" in recent years, as people look to gain health, wealth, a fulfilling relationship, or a promotion at work. If you are not familiar with maxim, it teaches that like attracts like, which is usually interpreted to mean

| High Consciousness — Aligned With True Self | Low Consciousness — Misaligned With True Self |
|---|---|
| Symptom free | Symptomatic |
| Feel connected and at peace | Feel disconnected and off-kilter |
| Clear mind | Cluttered mind |
| Higher level performance/you are on top of your game | Performance drops as mind gets busier |
| Life seems to flow | Life is an uphill struggle |
| Feel good about yourself & life | Don't feel good about yourself |
| Compassionate outlook | Negative or hostile outlook |
| Experience emotional stability | Experience emotional instability |
| Good things just seem to happen | Bad things seem to happen |
| Seeking solutions | Stuck in problems |
| High level of trust of intuition | Ignore intuition, tendency to over think everything |
| Decision making is easy and effective | Decision making is difficult and often turns out badly |

that if you think positive thoughts you will attract positive experiences into your life. What usually follows is that people go through a process of visualization or affirmations with a focus on positive thoughts. But if reports are anything to go by this often fails to materialize in people's lives. The approach isn't surprising because thinking is our default mode, so it would make sense that when introduced to a new concept we would naturally expect to filter it through our thinking channel.

However, if this approach isn't fruitful, what's going wrong? Rather than assuming that the law of attraction is not working because positive thoughts are not manifesting into that new house or job promotion, what if we entertain the idea that we are already creating our "reality" whether we are aware of it or not? Our "reality" comprises internal and external experiences. Our internal experience is what we feel and our external experience is what takes place in our environment, what shows up in our lives.

We live in a culture that conditions us to believe that life happens to us, that we adapt to circumstances and that we are, to a greater or lesser extent, victims of circumstance. This general view leads us to believe that we are passive observers of life, and while this does seem to match our five-sense reality or experience, it isn't particularly helpful as we aim to take charge of our health and take charge of our destiny. So, we need to turn this on its head and open up to the possibility that we are powerful creators and, rather than dealing with life as it happens we are creating life before it happens.

If we are contributing to the creation of our experience of reality what we need to know is what exactly contributes to this creation experience and what can we direct or affect. As we have seen from the Pygmalion effect, there is a circular causality at play where our beliefs and expectations impact our behavior and actions, which then affects what we experience. Life is perception, there is almost no absolute truth merely a series of perceptions. We imprint meaning and we filter out information based on our beliefs and conceptions of the world and ourselves. Our identity is a powerful driver for our behavior and though cognitive dissonance and confirmation bias we have a tendency to delete and distort the information that comes in through our senses so that it matches our conception of reality and our identity.

Our internal feeling experience is affected by our beliefs, behaviors, words, and thoughts. We transmit electromagnetic and possibly other subtle energies though our biofield, which exerts an influence on our experience. Like tuning a radio set into a particular frequency, we only receive the channel that we are tuned into, despite the fact all the other channels are still broadcasting at the same time. As we vibrate we are like human tuning forks, we resonate with certain "realities" and therefore it is these realities that we experience. If we are not vibrationally tuned-into these realities we simply don't experience them.

Are we in complete control of our level of vibration? No, we're not. There are things that lie beyond or outside are ability to direct, including our life lessons, which form part of our innate wiring; the vibration and energy of mass consciousness and the ebb and flow of energy and vibration that impacts the planet and the entire universe.

However, it is important for us to focus on what we can impact or affect. Our capability as transmitters of energy goes beyond the emotional energy we broadcast magnetically through our energy field. The biologist Rupert Sheldrake reported in his book, *The Sense Of Being Stared At,* a series of experiments to show that we transmit energy simply by looking and observing. Everything we place our attention upon we energetically "feed" and help to create. As we move through life we are moving through a vibrational energy soup and we everything we come into contact with receives our energetic imprint. Everything we focus our attention upon is influenced by our energetic transmission. This is something of a paradigm shift from the notion that we are victims of circumstance: as the cliché goes, "energy flows where attention goes."

## Practical Creation

The idea of us being vibrational beings tuning into different frequencies is all well and nice, but how do we harness this notion and take practical action in our everyday lives? The first step is to realize that:

*Everything you look at, think about, talk about, listen to, interact with, place your attention and intention upon, you energetically feed, reinforce, and breathe life into.*

Whatever you place your attention on, your intelligent body "thinks" is important, so the more attention you give something the more emotional feedback you will get, and the more intense that emotional feedback will be. Let's use a simple example: If you have, up until this point, had nothing more than a passing interest in football, there's a good chance that you don't experience any great emotion about football games. If you began to watch, read about players, get the views of pundits, talk to your friends about football, you'll find that your intelligent body responds by sending more emotion about football. You'll be more excited watching games, experience greater tension, and more disappointment if "your" team loses. Simply by directing your attention toward football you are teaching your intelligent body that football is important, and it responds by sending more emotion about football. This does not mean that your emotion is wrong or lies or is deceiving you in some way; it is always giving you feedback about your interaction with you environment and is always guiding you back to your true self. So changing your interaction with your environment will change your emotional experience.

What is evident is that we are impacting our emotional experience directly; it's simply not the case that emotions are completely beyond our control. Obviously there are things that grab our attention, things that we are interested in and passionate about. However, a significant amount of our emotion will be created as a result of where we place our attention and intention. This is what is meant by "energetically feeding" ideas and notions in the world around us. I literally mean that we breathe life into events and concepts. A significant aspect of our reality and how we create it comes about through focused intention and attention.

If you stop for a moment and review your current life and the journey you have taken to this point, you may begin to see the role you have played in creating this experience for yourself. If not, that's fine as well. It can require a significant shift in thinking to embrace the notion that the experience of life you are having is one in which you have played a major role in creating. This can be especially difficult if you dislike your life at the moment or feel that you have been dealt an unfair hand. It is however, important that you allow yourself to take responsibility from a space of empowerment, not blame. Empowerment is about taking responsibility for every aspect of yourself in order to move forward in a positive way. Blame is constrictive and negative; it will lead to a blockage of energy flow, negative emotions, and a likely increase in symptoms.

Everything that shows up in your life is there to serve you, to teach you in some way, to offer an opportunity—we could even go so far as to suggest that everything that shows up has been chosen by you at some level. This is not always obvious and can be difficult when our experience appears to be negative. However, when we understand that what we experience reflects our level of vibration it beings to make sense. If we truly have life lessons then we are likely to face experiences that we need to learn and grow from.

In order for us to be able to learn from our experience we need to step back, allow it to happen, remove any judgment and have an intention that we will integrate the learning. Whatever you are experiencing is a reflection of how you are choosing to experience your life. If you find that you are worried a lot of the time, it's not that life is worrying, it's that at some level you are choosing to experience life through the "lens" of worry. This is neither good not bad, right nor wrong, it is simply experience. When the experience seems unpleasant it is easy to dismiss as something undesirable that is happening to you. But if you want to redirect your experience to something more pleasant you have to understand that there is probably something in your current experience that is serving you—even if it that is simply having the experience of perceiving the world through the eyes of worry.

Start by opening up to the question, "What positive intention does this experience have for me? And, what does going through this experience enable me to do differently in the future?" Even if you don't have an answer, you are placing your attention and intention on finding an answer and that is the most important first step.

When I started to see the enormous role I was playing in the creation of my own experience and reality, it was really overwhelming. I could see there were a number of things happening in my life that I didn't want. Like a light bulb moment that offers a momentary glimpse to what is really going on, I could see that I was creating my experience, but I couldn't immediately see how to pull myself out of the cycle. I could sense my vibration and how my expectations and conceptions of my own identity were manifesting in my reality.

Much of what was contributing to my uncomfortable experiences was where I placed my attention, and this was affected by my unconscious expectations. I could see that there were unconscious "beliefs" that were impacting upon my behavior, outlook, approach, perspective, and ultimately expectation. I then had the realization that even though I couldn't immediately see how to pull myself out, the very fact that I had created one set of experiences meant that I could create a different set and these could be pleasant experiences that would serve my highest and best interest. So I set an intention that I would create experiences that were different and more pleasant, while still serving my highest and best interest.

To move forward with this idea of creation, we need to break it down into manageable chunks. The first step is to open up to the possibility that you are creating at least some of your experience—even if you don't have any idea how to change it. Creating your experience ranges from simple everyday interactions and exchanges through to bigger patterns that are present in your life. The good news is that we don't need to spend hours and hours unpicking your unconscious beliefs and conditioned patterns. You just need to begin by raising awareness of what is happening now and allow yourself to naturally align with your true self. You have incredible capacity to take charge of your life and personal sense of reality. Your default "factory" setting is to align with your true self, so you will natural drift towards higher consciousness, and even though we are facing challenging and changing times on this planet, the path forward involves simplifying our experience not complicating it. Trusting those deeper intuitions and feelings.

If you are used to feeling negative, it can feel like being stuck in a whirlwind of your own creation. That's okay! You don't have to know the way out: just follow these steps:

Develop your awareness for what you are placing your attention on, what you look at, think about, talk about, interact with. All these activities are literally energetic in nature. If you need to take one or two days to begin with to enable you to focus, put this in your schedule.

Place your attention, intention, words, thoughts, and actions on what you want to breathe life into, what you wish to experience, what you want to create. You will be amazed as you redirect your attention away from what you don't want towards what you do want, how much your life will change.

If you would like more structure to this, you can try the exercise below. There are three parts, which you can do in sequence or all at once, it's entirely up to you. Don't overload yourself, and make sure you give your full attention to each part.

PART I

1. Write down at least three things you want less of in your life. This could be anything from symptoms to a squeaky front door.

2. Review the last two to four weeks and think about how much attention you have given these things you want less of—write this down. This could include time spent thinking about, reading, talking about, etc.

3. As you look forward to the next two to four weeks, think about how you can remove your attention and energy from these things.

4. Replace the activities with those in Part 2.

PART 2

1. Write down at least three things you want more of in your life—these could be anything from a car to an expanded sense of self-awareness, to great success, to a life filled with love.

2. As you look forward for the next two to four weeks, how can you direct attention and energy into these things?

3. Can you imagine talking about them, thinking about them, reading, and researching?

4. Keep a check on yourself over the next month and make sure that you breathe life and energy into these things you want more of

5. If this part is a problem, don't worry, we have Part 3.

PART 3

1. Our aim is to raise our vibration—moving along the spectrum we talked about at the start of the book—and maintain a higher level so that the world we experience is one of a higher vibration.

2. In order to experience more love, joy, bliss, and compassion in your life you need to be "tuned-in" to that vibration.

3. What would it feel like in your body if your life was absolutely perfect: you are successful in every way, you have achieved everything you wanted, you are exactly the type of person you want to be, life could not be better.

You don't need to relate this to any actual events taking place, you don't need to know what those events are, you just need to feel in your body what it is like to already be there. Take as long as you need to imagine this now—this is the passion of the soul—don't think about this or force it, simply play with it and see where it takes you.

4. Once you have created that feeling, begin to create a feeling of gratitude for having such a perfect life. Again, take your time here.

5. Merge these feelings and notice what you feel in your body now. This may be very small to start, or may be an enormous feeling. Either way, your experience is unique and valid. Continue to practice and notice what happens as you do.

6. Memorize this new feeling. You are now more connected to your core frequency with a higher vibration. Practice creating and recreating this feeling as often as you can wherever you are. The more you can radiate this vibration the more your life will unfold on a similar frequency. Notice what happens in your daily life; how people are different with you, how circumstances seem different and maybe even turn out more favorably.

## The Road to Freedom

A general theme of this book is the notion of experiencing personal freedom through aligning and embracing more of who you are and who you can be. You are not fixed you are a flowing, evolving being. When you are free and aligned with your true self you will experience better health, deeper fulfillment, more happiness, and more harmonious relationships. When you are not aligned with your true self, you are constricted, your vibration drops and your life experience is far less desirable. In every aspect of life a removal of freedom is a cause of stress and distress; we seek connection with ourselves and each other, and so isolation and diminished freedom are punishing. The painful irony for many of us is that we are the ones who are removing our own freedom. We are not consciously constricting ourselves, rather our unconscious patterns and an outmoded sense of identity keep us locked on a path that deviates from the core of who we are. When we try to fit in, do the right thing, seek to be certain types of people, set expectations of how things should be, and set standards and ideals for achievement, we run the risk of shackling our own freedom—freedom to flow and experience ourselves in each moment as those moments arise. Most of the time we don't realize we are doing this, we are just running the old patterns.

Anytime you allow your mind to jump into the past or the future to think about or plan what you should do or say, you are preventing yourself from unfolding in the moment. We can get into a habit of confusing planning activities with planning how we should be. This is like when you are going to a social event and as well as planning how to get there, you start to think about how you should act, what you should do, who you should talk to and what you should say. When you do this your intelligent body will respond with discomfort and possibly symptoms. Your true self wants to *be*, it wants to experience life as it happens, it doesn't want to be shackled by the thinking egoic-mind deciding ahead of time what to say and do. Next time you notice yourself planning what to say and do, stop and pay attention to how your body feels and then remind yourself that you don't have to plan how to be, you just need to let yourself unfold, let yourself *be* . . . then notice how that feels.

Have you ever had a feeling of total freedom? Have you ever had the experience of walking to the top of a hill or mountain, pausing, looking all around, breathing deeply and having a sense of complete freedom? Whether you have or whether you haven't, I wonder if you can imagine for a moment, being stood on a mountain with your arms outstretched, breathing deeply and filling your lungs, the sun beating down on your face. As you look all around at the beauty of the planet you inhabit, you call out, "I am free, I am me, I am here, I am now. I am." Pause for a moment and allow yourself to feel that in your body now. Complete unbridled freedom with nothing to stop you or hold you back; freedom to be whoever you are whenever you like. You may notice the joy of allowing yourself to experience this or you may notice fear creeping in. Life can knock us and leave us wanting to build walls around ourselves rather than expose ourselves. Freedom to be exactly who we are may seem daunting and that's okay. The more you can remove judgment from all emotion and simply let it flow, the easier it will be to allow yourself to feel this expansive freedom, which is your birthright; it lies within you and is a part of who you are. If you were completely free to be experience all aspects of yourself, how would your life look? What would you do, who would you see, where would you go? Could you write that down, and would you want to?

There are two final exercises that you are invited to play with, both are designed to help you move towards experiencing more personal freedom from the inside out; meaning that our focus is experiencing a sense of freedom without having to manipulate external events.

This purpose of our first exercise is to release old patterns that may be keeping you stuck unknowingly in a low consciousness space of tension or pressure. Each of us has a tendency to put pressure on ourselves with expectations and worries without realizing. Habits form and we tune away from our feelings. Have you ever had the experience where you have stopped hearing some background noise, like road traffic in your house or place of work, and when someone new comes into that environment and they ask you what the noise is you have to recalibrate your ears to adjust and be able to hear it again? Our senses detect through difference or change, which means that if any of our senses are presented with a constant stimulus we lose our ability to detect it. This can happen with our emotions and moods as well. I first noticed this many years ago; I had set my sights on achieving a particular outcome and was applying significant internal pressure to myself without realizing. One day the pressure lifted and my internal sensations shifted, I felt lighter and happier, and it was only at that point I realized that I had been applying this pressure, which was causing internal stress and discomfort for a prolonged period of time. I had been in an ongoing state of stress and discomfort. I then began to see the pattern in my clients who were perpetually worrying, or putting pressure on themselves to be a certain type of person, or have certain types of experiences. This exercise will help shift those patterns that are ultimately constricting your freedom by helping you feel so you can spend more time in high consciousness and make better decisions and take more productive action.

We have discussed the idea that our thoughts and memories could potentially exist as fields of energy and information. The way I like to think of this is that our thoughts and memories are like a series of bubbles floating all around us. Do you remember being a kid and blowing bubbles? Some were big some were small and they could be floating all around your head and body. We could think of our thoughts and memories as being bubbles all around us. As we energetically feed these bubbles they get bigger and move closer to us. As we remove our attention from these bubbles they get smaller and move farther away. If we give something too much attention we can even find ourselves getting swallowed up by a bubble without realizing it. This first exercise will help you step back out of that bubble and withdraw your energy from it.

In practical terms, as you begin to work with this exercise you will become more conscious of how you feel and more able to shift and release unhelpful conditioned feeling states. Our health and happiness arise as a direct result of our interface with the world around us, so this process needs to be taken and applied in everyday life. Initially you will need to practice at home and then take what you have experienced into your daily life.

### The Exercise

Do this exercise for five to ten minutes every day but only do one part at a time. Take each part and spend five to seven days playing with it before moving on the next Part. You will probably find that there will be one or two Parts that are particularly relevant to you, so you might just want to focus on those.

In going through this exercise you may experience flashbacks from the past trying to hold on to the "old" you. You may experience sadness or other emotions, and may even experience memories that seem to jump into your mind. Allow yourself to notice and observe these experiences without getting stuck in them. Continue to let yourself flow and move, remember that everything you feel is transient as long as you allow yourself to feel it.

The aim is to feel into the body and learn from the experience by witnessing body sensations without labels or judgement. Start each part by focusing on your breathing, allowing yourself to develop a pattern of slower, deeper breathing, breathing in for a count of three and out for a count of five if that is comfortable; if not just breathe in a manner that feels comfortable in your body. Feel the breath. As you're doing this be aware of how your body feels. Allow tension to drop away from your body as your deeper breathing enables you to connect with your true self.

Once you have established the slower deeper breathing pattern focus on the feeling aspect of each Part. Create the feeling and notice whatever images and sounds arise. Simply notice the feelings of letting go and releasing and be aware of images that may arise. If images do arise allow yourself to pay attention to them and notice where they go, how they develop. You may feel yourself expand and feel constrictions, limitations, and walls fall away. You may also notice that your experience changes with each repetition of the exercise.

Having a conscious awareness of how you can feel will help when you go back to day-to-day life. The aim is to consciously choose how you approach and perceive life. As humans we notice and perceive through difference, so when we feel the same thing day to day we tend to become desensitized and miss how we are feeling. Practicing this exercise consistently will facilitate an increase in awareness of feeling states and help as you move towards conscious creation of day-to-day life.

PART I: WORRY

1. Feel into the potential that you don't have to worry about anything. That means entertain the idea in your feeling body that you never have to worry again. You are stepping out of the bubble of worry and letting it drift away and get smaller in the distance. It's as if, like the captain of the spacecraft at the start of the chapter, you have been given this knowledge. You now know deep in your core that you never have to worry again.

2. Allow yourself to fully embrace this idea; what does it feel like? Notice what you feel and where you feel it in the body. Notice the body sensations. Stay with those feelings and remember them. Breathe slowly and deeply and embrace these feelings, observing how they flow and move.

3. Finally, use the exercise when you approach worrisome areas or aspects of your life. By approaching an activity, task, place or person from a different state of consciousness and awareness you are likely to behave in a different way and experience a different outcome. The more

you develop awareness of your feeling state the better equipped you will become at understanding, acting on or changing the feeling state. Taking what you have practiced and applying it to your daily life is a crucial aspect of this exercise.

## PART 2: PRESSURE

1. Just as we did with Part 1, feel into the potential that you can remove all pressure from yourself, you don't have to achieve anything. Just like you have encountered a divine intervention that has implanted this new knowledge inside you that you do not have to achieve anything, you may want to have experiences in life and have outcomes, but all the pressure of having to achieve can dissolve away. Step out of the bubble and sense it float away.

2. Allow yourself to fully embrace this idea; what does it feel like? Notice what you feel and where you feel it in the body. Notice the body sensations. Stay with those feelings and remember them. Breathe slowly and deeply and embrace these feelings, observing how they flow and move.

3. Finally, take this into "real life" and identify where and when you place pressure on yourself. Practice recreating your pressure-free state of consciousness and be curious about how you approach life and how your outcomes change.

## PART 3: DOING THINGS IN A CERTAIN WAY

1. Feel into the potential that you can let go of the idea that things need to be done a certain way. This could be expectations of activities, tasks or people, or the idea that things have to happen or be done in a certain way or at a certain time.

2. Simply embrace the idea of letting go and notice what that feels like in the body. Stay with those feelings and remember them. Breathe slowly and deeply and embrace these feelings while observing their flow.

3. Finally, use this exercise when you approach these areas or aspects of your life. Notice when you are beginning to

approach new situations from the perspective that things have to happen in a certain way (or at a certain time), and allow yourself to practice this part of releasing this need. Notice how you feel as you practice this. The fixation that things have to happen in a certain way is a product of the egoic mind, not the true self. Your true self is flexible and free and can deal with whatever happens. Use this part in daily life when you notice yourself fixating on doing things in a specific way.

PART 4: BEING A CERTAIN TYPE OF PERSON

1. Feel into the potential that you can let go of having to be a certain way or a certain type of person. Open up to the idea that you can simply be who you are without constriction or definition. As our identities begin to shift it can be helpful to simply observe and be curious as to who you might be rather than trying to define yourself by who you have been.

2. Feel how this feels in the body. Stay with these feelings and remember them. Breathe slowly and deeply and embrace these feelings.

3. Reflect on life in general and identify specific areas where you can recognize that you are trying to be a certain way or trying to create a certain type of impression. There could be all sorts of reasons for this, all primarily related to fitting in, conforming, and being concerned with other people's views and impressions of you.

4. Finally, use the exercise when you approach these areas or aspects of your life. Be conscious of times when you are trying to portray an image or yourself, or when you are trying to affect other people's impressions or thoughts about you; this is the time to use this part in your daily life. By approaching an activity, task, place or person from a different state of consciousness and awareness you are likely to behave in a different way and experience a different outcome. The more you develop awareness of your feeling state the better equipped you will become at understanding, acting on or changing the feeling state.

PART 5: RESPONSIBILITY

1. Feel into the potential that you can release all responsibility that is not directly associated with yourself. Release the need to frequently or constantly rescue people.

2. Allow yourself to fully embrace this idea; what does it feel like? Notice what you feel and where you feel it in the body. Notice the body sensations. Stay with these feelings and remember them. Breathe slowly and deeply and embrace these feelings, observing how they flow and move.

3. Reflect on life in general and identify specific areas where you are taking on responsibility for other people and this is leading to a buildup of tension inside your body. Remember that the more responsibility you take, the more you try to rescue, help, and look after other people where they should be looking after themselves, the more this will radiate out of your energy field and the more people will seek to have you rescue them.

5. Allow yourself to practice the first three steps in relation to each area where you are taking too much responsibility for others and facilitating their disempowerment.

6. Finally, use the exercise when you approach these areas or aspects of your life.

PART 6: NOTHING MATTERS

1. Finally, allow yourself to feel into the potential that nothing matters and that everything is fine. While this may seem extreme because you may assume that there are always going to be things in life that matter, being able to create a feeling state that all is well and nothing matters is truly freeing. The idea is that you are free to be you, to experience a state of high consciousness without being stuck to false notion or ideas. This step brings together all of the others. Stay with these feelings and remember them. Breathe slowly and deeply and embrace these feelings.

2. Notice how that feels. If there are any sensations of discomfort or tension allow yourself to simply notice.

3. Finally, use the exercise when you approach life in gen-

eral, when you notice that you are becoming fixated and tension is building in the body. By gently reminding yourself that nothing really matters, all is well, and that everything is simply experience, you are removing judgment and allowing energy to flow. As you move through your daily life some things will matter to you more than others, as you practice this part you will be better equipped to discern what really matters and why.

Remember, what we are doing with each part is feeling into potential. This exercise is not simply about trying to overlay a new feeling in order to avoid discomfort. The purpose is for us to begin to see that we are not controlled by outside events and that everything is fluid and flexible. To visit a notion from quantum theory, everything that can exist does exist and the potential is in this moment. Reality is our conception, not something fixed. Our experience of life does not have to be fixed; it can be changed in line with our highest and best interest. We can make these changes ourselves.

The final exercise in this chapter is to look at what do you want, what you wish to experience? This is your time to step up and create the life you want. Forget who you have been and open up to who you could be. Do you dare to dream?

1. Set some time aside when you will be able to relax and write without being disturbed. Get a paper and pen ready.

2. Write down what you want and what you wish to experience. These are experiences and potential directions in which to move or be guided, rather than absolute goals that are fixed and detailed. In attaining and creating our flow, we want to set intention without forcing or defining goals. If you find that nothing comes then put the pen and paper to one side and revisit this exercise at a later date.

3. If, however, you do find that ideas begin to flow freely, then allow yourself to be detailed or vague, stay out of the mind, and steer clear of boundaries and limits. Allow yourself to open up to your deepest heartfelt desires and write them down. You could write down exactly how you would like your life to be, or simply experiences you would like to have.

4. You may want to approach this exercise from the perspective that you are starting over or starting afresh, where anything is possible with no limits or boundaries, almost as if this is your intention for a happy fulfilled life.

5. Once you have finished, read through what you have written and notice what you feel.

6. Re-write your document so everything reads in the present tense as if you are currently doing the things you wish to experience, e.g. "I am doing . . .," "I feel great as I . . ." As you re-read the document what feelings do you notice with the document worded in the present tense? If there are any elements that do not resonate with you remove them

7. Type up this document and save it on your computer. Set an intention that you will allow yourself to flow towards this life or these activities if this is within your highest and best interest.

8. Revisit the document as frequently as you like to review your development and direction of flow.

As you revisit what you have written you will begin to notice that you are creating your life, you are experiencing more of what you want and that you are opening up to more of who you can be. Your self awareness will grow and your confidence and esteem will blossom as you see the impact you can have on your own life. You are now taking responsibility for yourself and have given up blaming anything or anyone outside of yourself, you recognize your role in the creation of your experience of reality. This is your time!

# A Final Thought

LET ME CONGRATULATE YOU ON COMPLETING THIS BOOK! IF you have created the time for yourself to try on the theory and play with the exercises, you have done magnificently well! The next step is to begin to practice implementing the principles and practices in your daily life. The more you practice, the more your life will change for the better. It takes a lot of courage to go against the stream of conventional thinking, to do something that challenges you to go deeper to find out who you really are and what you are really capable of. On the surface, many of these ideas may seem quite simple, but implementation can be like peeling away layers of the old programming and conditioning that have clouded your true self.

This book offers a fresh perspective on many aspects of health and well-being, which can take a while to sink in and fully absorb. I frequently have clients say to me that even though they've heard me say the same things over and over for a period of time, it has taken that time period before they really "get it." There is a difference between an intellectual understanding and a deep body appreciation. Being able to fully understand something to the point that it can impact at a deep level and help in creating lasting change can take time and practice. This book is intended to offer more than intellectual stimulation or interest; the intention is that it is the beginning of or a part of your journey of awakening to your true self and experience of health and well-being.

Before you move on from the ideas presented here, I encourage you to work on consolidating what you have learned here first. The thinking mind has a tendency to want novelty, which is not a bad thing, but this tendency can sometimes lead us to miss opportunities that are available to us. So I would suggest that you go through the book several times, and if you feel drawn to it, to include the chapters and exercises you might have skipped through, or to do the ones that you feel you had not given sufficient practice to once again, and even to repeat those that worked for you. You might be surprised how this commitment to finding a deeper view by means of repetition can bring about insights you may have only glimpsed the first time round.

You are also likely to find that completely fresh understandings arise when you repeat your reading and practice of the material. There are so many distractions in our daily lives that it is likely you might have missed some important and helpful details the first time you encountered this information. But be prepared for some resistance to repetition; the thinking mind often wants to move on because it subconsciously knows it has skipped over some details that are threatening to it. So repetition is part of the new courage you are learning. You are becoming more willing to let go of old thinking and habit patterns, and so some resistance will be part of that process. Be gentle with yourself if you sense this resistance, and come back to the material when you feel ready. This book is always at hand, so there is no need to rush. Even if you should move on to other teachings you might find that occasionally you are reminded of something you had encountered here. When that happens, give yourself the gift of returning to this material to immerse yourself in whatever aspect of it feels right for you at that time.

You have the capacity to make a significant difference to your health and the quality of your life. You don't have to continually seek answers outside of yourself—what you have read here will guide you back home, back to yourself.

The theory, principles, and practices outlined in this book have been developed over many years and not only have I honed and fine-tuned them with my clients in my clinical practice, I have used and still use them in my own life. It's over to you now; when you make that commitment to yourself and believe in your own ability to heal yourself, you will begin to see and feel yourself take great strides.

Enjoy the journey!

# READING LIST

Borrell-Carrióo, F., Suchman, A. L., & Epstein, R. M. (2004). The Bio-psychosocial Model 25 Years Later: Principles, Practice, and Scientific Enquiry. *Annals of Family Medicine,2*(6), 576–582. Retrieved from http://www.ncbi.nlm.nih.gov/pmc/articles/PMC1466742/

Brain & Behaviour Research Foundation. (From The Quarterly January 2016). The Biology of Emotions. Retrieved from https://bbrfoundation.org/discoveries/the-biology-of-emotions.

Calver, L. A., Barrie. J ., Stokes, B. J., & and Isbister, G. K. (2009). The Dark Side of the Moon. *Medical Journal Of Australia*. August 2009, 191 (11) 692–694.

Childre, D. & Martin, M. (1999). *The HeartMath Solution: Proven Techniques For Developing Emotional Intelligence*. London, Piatkus Books.

Cornelius, R. R. (1996). *The Science of Emotion: Research & Tradition in the Psychology of Emotion*. Princeton, NJ: Prentice Hall.

Cowie, R. (2015). The Enduring Basis of Emotional Episodes: Towards a Capacious Overview. *Affective Computing and Intelligent Interaction (ACII)*, 2015 International Conference, 98–104. IEEE.

Dalgleish, T. (2004). The Emotional Brain. *Nature Reviews: Neuroscience, 5*. 2004 July 5 (7), 583–589. Retrieved from http://www-psych.stanford.edu/~knutson/ans/dalgleish04.pdf

Damasio, A. (2000). *The Feeling of What Happens: Body and Emotions in the Making of Consciousness*. London: Vintage.

Damasio, A. (2005). Feeling Our Emotions. *Scientific American*. April 2005. Retrieved from http://www.scientificamerican.com/article/feeling-our-emotions/

Dinan, T. G. & Cryan, J. C. F. (2012). Regulation of the Stress Response by the Gut Microbiota: Implications for Psychoneuroendocrinology. *Psychoneuroendocrinology, 37*(9), 1369–78. doi: 10.1016/j.psyneuen.2012.03.007. Epub 2012 Apr 5

Felitti, V. J., *et al.* (1998). Relationship of childhood abuse and household dysfunction to many of the leading causes of death in adults. *American Journal of Preventative Medicine, 14*(4), 245–258.

Forrester, M. (2013). How DNA is Reprogrammed by Words and Frequencies. *Waking Times.* Retrieved from http://www.wakingtimes.com/2013/08/05/how-dna-is-reprogrammed-by-words-and-frequencies/

Gefter, A. (2016). The Case Against Reality. *The Atlantic.* Retrieved from http://www.theatlantic.com/science/archive/2016/04/the-illusion-of-reality/479559/

Gilman, R. (1984). Memory and Morphogenetic Fields. *Context Institute.* Retrieved from http://www.context.org/iclib/ic06/gilman2/

Gratrix, N. (2016, March 26). Healing Emotional Trauma Part I: How Does Our Childhood Biography Become Our Biology?. Retrieved from http://www.nikigratrix.com/healing-emotional-trauma-part-1-how-does-our-biography-become-our-biology/

Herremans, D. (2008, October 22). The World's First Global Peace Intention Experiment. *Natural News.* Retrieved from http://www.naturalnews.com/024576_violence_experiments_death.html

Hill, A. (2007, September 2). Cancer Warning for Stressed-Out Men. *The Observer.* Retrieved from https://www.theguardian.com/uk/2007/sep/02/health.gender

Immordino-Yang, M. H. (2016). *Emotions, Learning, & the Brain: Exploring The Educational Implications Of Affective Neuroscience.* New York: W. W. Norton & Company, Inc.

Jackson, M. (2014). Evaluations the Role of Hans Selye in the Modern history of Stress. *Stress, Shock, and Adaptation in the Twentieth Century* (Chapter 1). Retrieved from http://www.ncbi.nlm.nih.gov/books/NBK349158/

Johnston, E. & Olson, L. (2015). *The Feeling Brain: The Biology and & Psychology of Emotions.* New York: W. W. Norton & Company, Inc.

Kirmayer, L. J., Groleau, D., Looper, K. J., & Doa, M. D. (2004). Explaining Medically Unexplained Symptoms. *Canadian Journal of Psychiatry*, October 2004, 49 (10), 663–672. doi: 10.1177/070674370404901003. Retrieved from http://cpa.sagepub.com/content/49/10/663.abstract

Lewis, M., Haviland-Jones, J. M., & Feldman Barrett, L. (Editors) (2008). *Handbook of Emotions*, Third Edition. New York, The Guildford Press.

Maes, M. (2013). Inflammatory and Oxidative and Nitrosative Stress Cascades as New Drug Targets in Myalgic Encephalomyelitis and Chronic Fatigue Syndrome. *Modern Trends in Pharmacopsychiatry, 28,* 162–74. doi: 10.1159/000343982. Epub 2013 Feb 27.

Maté, G. (2013). *When The Body Says No: Exploring The Stress-Disease Connection.* London: John Wiley & Sons.

Maté, G. (2016, November 16). How to Build a Culture of Good Health. *Yes Magazine.* Retrieved from http://www.yesmagazine.org/issues/good-health/gabor-mate-how-to-build-a-culture-of-good-health-20151116

McCraty, R. (2015). *Science Of The Heart: Exploring The Role of The Heart in Human Performance Volume 2* (ebook). Boulder, CA, HeartMath Institute.

McTaggart, L. (2001). *The Field.* London: Element (HarperCollins).

Myers, W. (2016, May 14). The Emotional Causes of Cancer. Retrieved from https://liveto110.com/the-emotional-causes-of-cancer/

Nierenberg, C. (2016, May 20). The Science of Intuition: How To Measure 'Hunches' and 'Gut Feelings'. *Live Science.* Retrieved from http://www.livescience.com/54825-scientists-measure-intuition.html

Papez, J. W. (1937). A Proposed Mechanism Of Emotion. *Archives Of Neurology & Psychiatry, 38*(4), 725–743.

Pert, C. B. (1997). *Molecules Of Emotion: Why You Feel The Way You Feel.* London: Simon & Schuster UK Ltd.

Pert, C. B. (2006). *Everything You Need To Know To Feel Good.* London, Hay House UK Ltd.

Pontin, J. (2014). The Importance of Feelings. *Technology Review.* Retrieved from https://www.technologyreview.com/s/528151/the-importance-of-feelings/

Popova, M. (2015). The Science of Stress and how Our Emotions Affect Our Susceptibility to Burnout and Disease. *Brain Pickings.* Retrieved from https://www.brainpickings.org/2015/07/20/esther-sternberg-balance-within-stress-emotion/

Prinz, J. (2003). Emotions embodied (pdf). (Penultimate version of chapter in R. Solomon (Ed.) Thinking about Feeling. New York: OUP 2003). Retrieved from http://subcortex.com/PrinzEmotionsEmbodied.pdf.

Rother, S. (2004). *Spiritual Psychology: The Twelve Primary Life Lessons.* Poway, CA: Lightworker Publications.

Schwartz, G. E. R. (2007). *The Energy Healing Experiments: Science Reveals Our Natural Power to Heal.* New York: Atria Books.

Schwartz, G. E. R. & Russek, L. G. S. (1999). *The Living Energy Universe: A Fundamental Discovery That Transforms Science & Medicine.* Charlottesville, VA: Hampton Roads Publishing Company Ltd.

Selye, H. (1978). *The Stress of Life* (Revised Edition). New York, McGraw-Hill Book Company.

Servan-Schreiber, D. (2005). *Healing Without Prozac & Freud: Natural Approaches To Curing Stress, Anxiety & Depression.* London: Rodale.

Sheldrake, S. (1989). *The Presence Of The Past.* London: HarperCollins.

Sheldrake, S. (1999). *Dogs That Know When Their Owners Are Coming Home and Other Unexplained Powers of Animals.* London: Arrow Books.

Sheldrake, S. (2003). *The Sense Of Being Stared At and Other Aspects of the Extended Mind.* London: Arrow Books.

Szabo, S., Tache, Y., & Somogyi, A. (2012). The Legacy Of Hans Selye And The Origins Of Stress Research: A Retrospective 75 years After His Landmark 'Letter' To The Editor Of *Nature. Stress, 15*(5), 472–478.

Tomas, C., Newton, J., & Watson, S. (2013). A Review of Hypothalamic-Pituitary-Adrenal Axis Function in Chronic Fatigue Syndrome. ISRN Neuroscience. Sep 30, 2013, 784520. doi: 10.1155/2013/784520. eCollection 2013. Retrieved from http://www.ncbi.nlm.nih.gov/pubmed/24959566.

Twisk, F. N. (2014). The Status of and Future Research into Myalgic Encephalomyelitis and Chronic Fatigue Syndrome: The Nedd of Accurate Diagnosis, Objective Assessment, and Acknowledging Biological and Clinical Subgroups. *Frontiers In Physiology.* 2014 Mar 27, 5, 109. doi: 10.3389/fphys.2014.00109. eCollection 2014.

Wade, D. T. & Halligan, P. W. (2004). Do Biomedical models Of Illness Make For Good Healthcare Systems. *British Medical Journal, 329,* 398–401.

Wang, Y. & Kasper, L. H. (2014). The Role Of Microbiome in Central Nervous System Disorders. *Brain, Behaviour and Immunity, 38,* 1–12. doi: 10.1016/j.bbi.2013.12.015

Watzlawick, P., Weakland, J. Fisch, R. (1974). Change: Principles of Problem Formation & Problem Resolution. New York: W. W. Norton & Company, Inc.

Wolkin, J. (2015, August 14). Meet Your Second Brain: The Gut. *Mind-*

*ful*. Retrieved from http://www.mindful.org/meet-your-second-brain-the-gut/

Wolynn, M. (2016, May 19). It Didn't Start with You: how Inherited Family Trauma Shapes Who We Are. *Science and Nonduality*. Retrieved from https://www.scienceandnonduality.com/an-excerpt-from-it-didnt-start-with-you-how-inherited-family-trauma-shapes-who-we-are-and-how-to-end-the-cycle-viking-april-2016-by-mark-wolynn.

# INDEX

Note: Italicized page locators refer to figures; tables are noted with *t*.